I0022816

ENERGY

MINDSET

TRANSFORM

YOUR LIFE

Joyce A. Pellegrini

Pellegrini Publications

DISCLAIMER

This book is not intended to provide medical advice, or in any way attempt to practice medicine. It is not intended to replace personal medical care from a licensed health care practitioner. Doing anything recommended or suggested in this book must be done at your own risk.

DEDICATION

This book is dedicated to my brother, Perry Pellegrini, who fought so hard to beat cancer but lost and left this world on his 46th birthday.

Perry and I had a very combative relationship. However, if one of us was in need we could always count on each other 100% without question or hesitation. The moment I heard his diagnosis of 7 months to live I packed up my 2-seater car with Rocky, my dog, and was at his house within 24 hours from Florida to Chicago. I had enough fight in me for both of us. I was going to help him win this battle if it was the last thing I did!

Perry answered the door and said, "I knew you would come", as we cried in each other's arms. Perry died 7 months from his diagnosis

There is not a day that goes by that I do not think of you and I feel your presence when I am in need especially while riding my Harley.

We had so many identical personality traits and as I watched him take his last breath I realized how precious life was and not to be taken for granted. The moment he was gone I vowed to myself that this will not happen to me. I will do whatever it takes to live a healthy and vibrant life.

Being one of Perry's care givers educated me on how destructive it is to hold on to emotional strife. Emotional and mental stress will break down the immune system. His death revealed the importance of paying attention to your body. Perry had many signs but did not listen until he felt and said, "I feel like I am dying!" For this reason, his death was senseless to me.

Perry, I see you whole, at peace, no pain, and holding court with Dad and the rest of our departed loved ones.

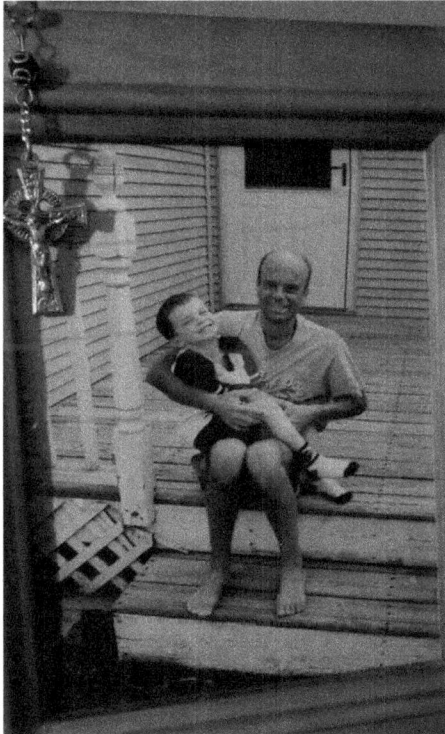

Perry with 5-year-old son Sean a few months before he passed.

I love and miss you and I dedicate my life's work in memory of you! May you continue to watch over all of us and truly rest in peace little brother.

Life is not a dress rehearsal. It is not too late to STOP and change the course of your life and health which, in turn, will change the course of your family's future.

My mission in life is to live life filled with passion, purpose, and **FULL THROTTLE ENERGY**!

ACKNOWLEDGMENTS

I have worked with so many amazing holistic health and wellness professionals that have shared their gifts throughout the years. Filled with gratitude that they shared their wisdom, energy, written words, lectures, love, and healing touch. Their bright white light has not been forgotten.

- Sue Mislich Dercole – Body Builder, Mentor, Drill Sergeant, Motivator

- Virginia Dassler – Herbology & Kinesiology

- Dr. Bill Nelson – Creator of SCIO Technology

- Gage Tarrant – SCIO Master Biofeedback Instructor

- Kathy Heaverlo – SCIO Practitioner & Mentor

- Ursula Kaiser – BFF – Educator, Mentor, and Stage 4 Cancer Survivor 18 Years & Thriving

- Louise Hay – Thought Leader

- Barbara Dekker Ellis - SCIO Regional Manager

- Debbie Thurman Strawder – SCIO Practitioner

- Jimmy Mack – Liquid Fish Creator - Healer

- Diane Marie Billman – Human Scale, Access Consciousness & Intuitive

- Liz Mason – Certified Donna Eden Practitioner, LMT

- Lisa Hein - Spiritual Mentor

- Bonnie Bateman – LMT Extraordinaire

- Ilana – Voice Printing/Light Therapist

- Paige Clarke – Holistic Approach to Health & Wellness Educator

- Dr. Hongjian He – Oriental Medicine Doctor

- Dr. Joshua Plant – Biochemist Zija Formulator

- Grand Master Dennis Kelly - Chi Kung Instructor

- Natalie Ledwell – Mind Movies

- Dr. Hilda Maldonado – Functional Medicine Holistic Approach & Thyroid Specialist

- Lani Reagan – Intuitive Life Coach & Healer

- Tiffany Robles – Accountability Partner, Mindfulness Mentor, and Owner Koei-Kan Martial Arts Academy

- Isaac Michalov – Soul Brother and a great male role model in my life. You have blessed me with your loving energy. I look forward to growing old together. Thank you for sharing your knowledge, heart, family, and home when I'm in California.

- Joel Bauer - a very special THANK YOU. It is because of you that I have been inspired to write 4 books and 2 Programs over a short period of time. He cracked my heart wide open in 2010 and through his processes gave me the strength and courage to move past my own self-limiting beliefs. This book from within was inspired by Joel to take one of my passions in life and inspire others that it is never too late to BE – DO – HAVE the life you were meant to live.

I will be forever grateful to all my amazing Mentors and Practitioners in my life.

CONTENTS

1 ENERGY

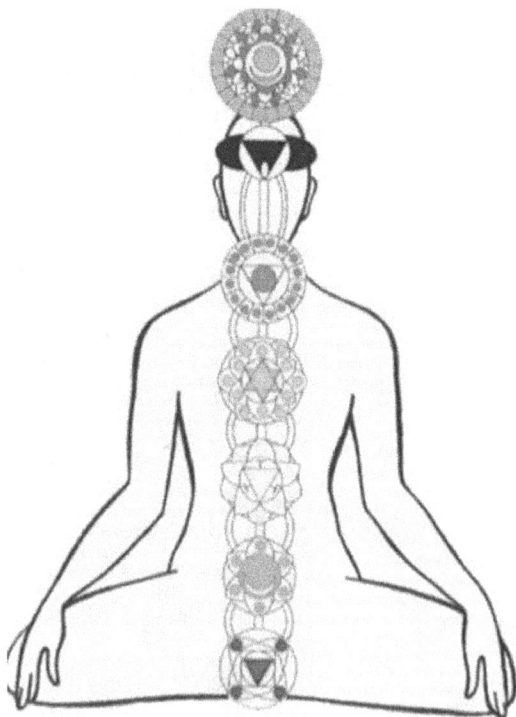

Crown - Spiritual

3rd Eye - Perception

Throat - Expression

Heart - Love

Solar Plexus - Power

Sacral - Sex

Root - Survival

The **energy** of a **body** or system because of its position in an electric, magnetic, or gravitational field.

My Journey of Awareness and Enlightenment is to share how I had to drastically shift my ENERGY and MINDSET from the following list of life lessons that has brought me here today.

- Forgiveness

- Truth

- Authenticity

- Effective Communication

- Anger/Hatred

- Depression

- Limiting Beliefs

- Lack of Passion and Purpose

- Exhaustion Workaholic

- Clarity Lost

- No Joy or Happiness

I could not forgive my father. I was afraid to speak my truth. I was hiding my true self and not being authentic. I had no idea how to communicate effectively. Had suppressed anger and hatred. Became a workaholic and felt depressed. I believed everything I heard from my father that kept me in a lack of believing in myself. Passion and purpose was fueled in unhealthy ways. No clarity of where I wanted to go.

Realized I had no joy or happiness in my personal life. Hit Corporate burnout in 2001. I walked away from everything I knew to be true! I had been addicted to sleeping pills for 12 years and decided to fire my doctor. That day I made a conscious choice to learn everything I could about healing my mind, body, and spirit naturally.

A few years later, I met Barbara Dekker at the Ritz Carlton with Ursula Kaiser my BFF and wellness coach.

Ursula was told over 18 years ago that she had 3 months to live. Really? Back then, there was no internet. Ursula began to read many books on how to detox her body. She found a holistic cancer treatment center in Mexico and began the process of detoxing her mind, body, and spirit. Ursula had been a vegan most of her adult life, never drank or smoked, was very active, and no body fat. She took care of herself so why did she get cancer?

Ursula believes that the stress of a law suit that lasted many years broke down her inner spirit and immune system. However, she had the grit and determination not to allow either one of them to break her. The human spirit and the mind can do amazing things. Ursula now lectures and shares her story to inspire
others never to give up hope that all things are possible.

It is my belief that the human body is an amazing computer system. When you eat core nutrition, drink good water, positive attitude, laughter, low stress, we can change the course of any diagnosis or health issue. We are lucky to be in a world that information is just a click away. However, please work with your Doctor through your health and wellness journey.

Some history of my being stressed to the max, unhealthy, and miserable. Back in 2004, Ursula introduced me to Barbara Dekker, a Stress Management Coach, who changed the course of my life the day we met!

Barbara's sessions educated her clients how stress affected their mind, body, and spirit. The technology used was an energy/frequency machine that used quantum physics. I was so intrigued with the information I followed her home and had my first biofeedback session. I was blown away by the coaching session. The information was 100% accurate. I even felt the subtle energy running through my body.

I wanted to know more about how ENERGY can become stagnate in the body. I became aware of how destructive my negative thought patterns affected me as well.

Barbara spent time sharing my mental and emotional stressors to exactly where my blockages were in that moment.

My husband and I decided to divorce in 2003 and was heartbroken, devastated, felt abandoned, and betrayed. The report stated betrayal, abandoned, depression, resentment, anger, religious conflict, resistance to change, desire for things to be different, forgiveness, to name a few. Can you relate to this story?

I must admit, I felt every emotion deeply which pushed out suppressed tears as she began to balance and shift my energy. After my fourth session, I was so impressed with the technology, took a leap of faith, and purchased equipment/program and never looked back.
I began my journey healing my mind, body, and spirit over

15 years ago. This was health no accident. I was ready and pumped to embark on a new career. I was the most stressed person I knew so it was time for the healer to heal thyself.

This biofeedback program stated the exact stuck emotions I had since early childhood. The truth of it all shocked me into action. Time to make necessary life style changes which made all the difference.

Today I rarely get sick. My immune system is strong. Even my thyroid Doctor said, "your blood work is amazing you better be saving money you will live a very long life." Great report to get from Dr. Drucker. It was due to reducing my stress, cleaning up diet, stopped negative thought patterns, no drama, and my personal goal is to live well pass 100 years of age.

STRESS is the number one silent killer. When we do not address our daily stress, it continues to break down our immune system and months or years later we are diagnosed with some form of disease or health issue.

We are 100% energy and act like magnets. When we have negative thoughts, we vibrate at a specific frequency. When we resonate at a low frequency it is matched. When our energy is high and positive all things are possible. It is really that easy. Why do we make life so difficult?

An example, I use to attract angry men to me. I was doing an energy session with Bob Kilpatrick and he said, "You can only resonate what you are." Wow, I did not like that answer and thought about it all week. As I began to go deeper and reflect I realized my dad was angry, mom's anger suppressed, the rest of my siblings had some anger issues, and so did I! My light bulb went on and realized my anger was so suppressed due to lack of communication skills. I was unable to communicate properly which was the reason why I was a chronic insomniac. I had no peace, joy, or happiness. Have you ever felt like that? Unspoken words will kill you!

Purchasing technology and doing sessions on myself daily I saved my life. I am living proof of my own work. Learning about my food sensitivities and the correct thyroid product made the difference. The picture below was 9 years ago, 194 pounds.

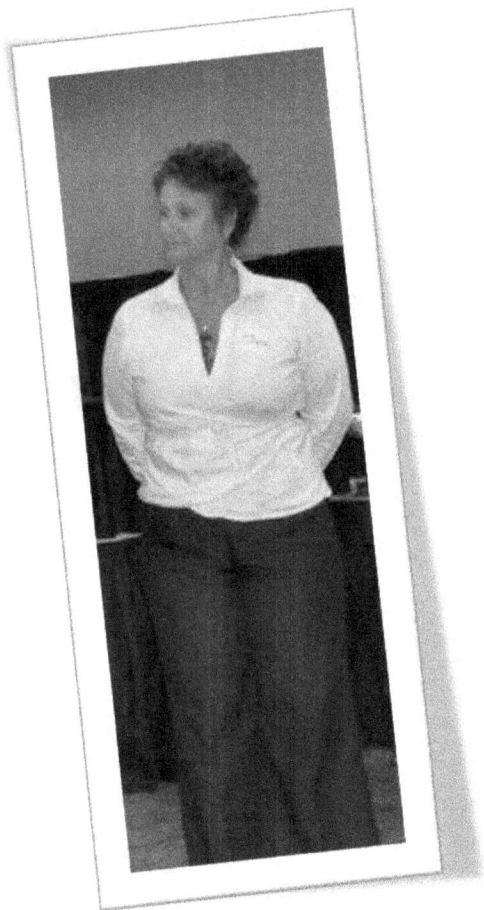

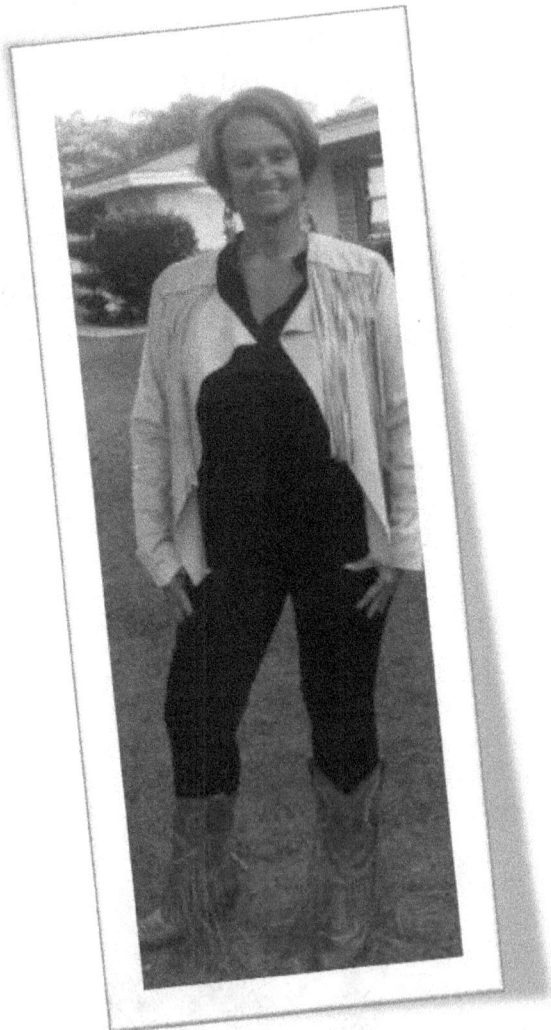

Above, 2018, 155 pounds. I feel and look better than I did 20 years ago. That is my wish for you.

It is never too late to live your life by design and not by default. Thanks Joel Bauer. I embrace that statement daily and hope you will too.

I am not a Doctor and my journey of awareness is to share just that, my journey. I highly suggest you do your own due diligence on the body's electric, ENERGY. I recommend Authors below to take your knowledge deeper.

- Nikola Tesla – Pure Genius

- Dr. Joe Dispenza – Breaking the Habit of Being You

- Masaru Emoto

- Eckhart Tolle

- Gregg Braden

- Dan Millman

- Donna Eden

I have performed 1000s of sessions on clients, family, and friends. It is so important to manage your stress, learn how it affects your mind, body, and spirit, implement easy action steps, and shift your energy now. Understanding the body's electric, ENERGY, is the key to your vitality.

My goal is to touch those that crave something better with guaranteed results when you take action. It is now time to live your life full throttle so you can BE - DO – HAVE all that you desire.

Balance Your Energy for Vitality

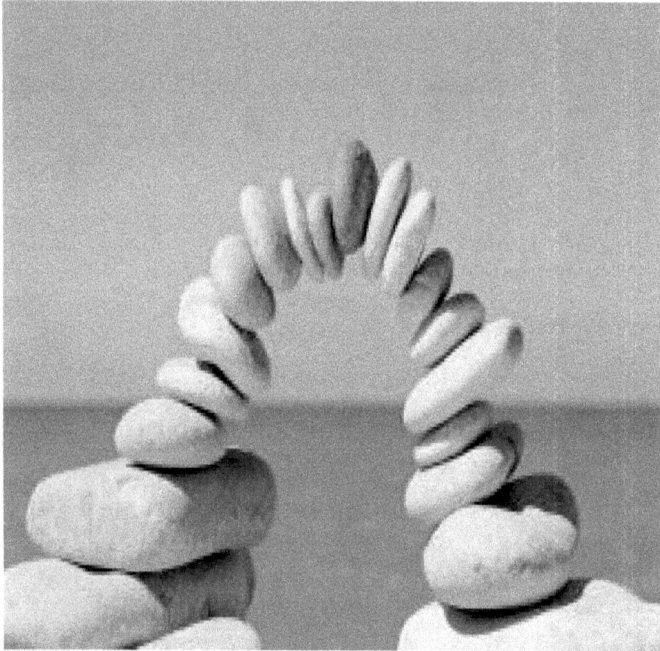

Mantras I Live By

"What you think about you bring about."

"What you resist persists."
Law of Attraction

FEAR
False Evidence Appearing Real

Health Goes Where Energy Flows

Seek the gift in all that happens and you shall find peace from within!

5 – 4 – 3 – 2 – 1
5 Second Rule by Mel Robbins
Shift Your Energy

EMBRACE
Your Body's Electric

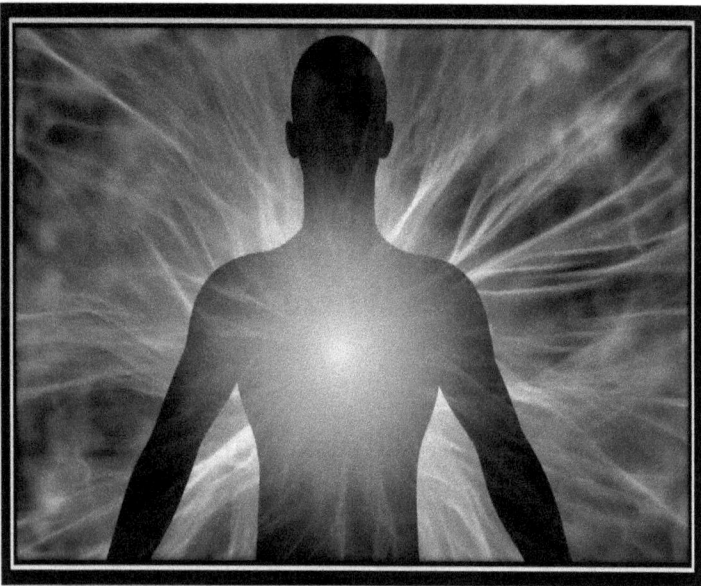

2 MINDSET

What is mindset and why it matters?

Your mindset plays a critical role in how you cope with life's challenges. In life, a growth mindset can contribute to greater achievement and increased effort. When facing a problem such as trying to find a new job, people with growth mindsets show greater resilience.

Your thoughts are very important. I was having a very hard time with negative thoughts and self-hatred many years ago! When I left Corporate America in 2001, I was mentally and emotionally burnt out. I was walking with a friend and she checked me by saying "Joyce do you hear yourself talking?"

"You have not said one good thing about yourself." BAM right between the eyes.

Ursula Kaiser also made the same statement and gave me "The Secret" Law of Attraction DVD to watch but for six months it just sat on my night stand. One morning, at 5 a.m., another sleepless night was the day of reckoning. I put that DVD in my lap top and cried throughout the entire movie. The message hit me so profoundly.

I would start my morning watching that DVD for the next 30 days. Each morning a new message was delivered which I missed the day before. It took me a month until I could wrap my head around the concept of "What you think about you bring about" and "What you resist persists."

I had no idea how negative I truly was about my own life and the terrible choices I made. I had no one to blame but myself, because I did not listen to that gut feeling. Do you allow your decisions to be made from your heart or head? I projected a positive attitude to everyone I met, but down deep to my core I had self-hatred. Why? It was after I left my executive career, 9/11 happened, and I was unable to get a job. I beat myself up daily over my "failures". A major take-away was…

HEALTH GOES WHERE ENERGY FLOWS!

This statement resonated so deeply within me. It was the day I began to stop degrading myself. I pulled out my tools that

I had from the past and began to create positive action steps to create the life I was meant to live.

I began to socialize with other healers and found Sharon

Kistler who organized a spiritual group named the Amazing Women Network. I went to my first meeting and we created a VISION BOARD which I have today in my office. I really enjoyed the process and it shifted my energy and I began to DREAM AGAIN. Through this process I realized how beaten I felt, stopped dreaming, and gave up. My mom said to me often:

"You are such a DREAMER you better marry a millionaire!"

Do you have family or friends that joke about your dreams? I sure hope not! If you do STOP telling them your goals and connect with like-minded individuals that will lift you up and assist you in reaching all you desire. It is imperative for success.

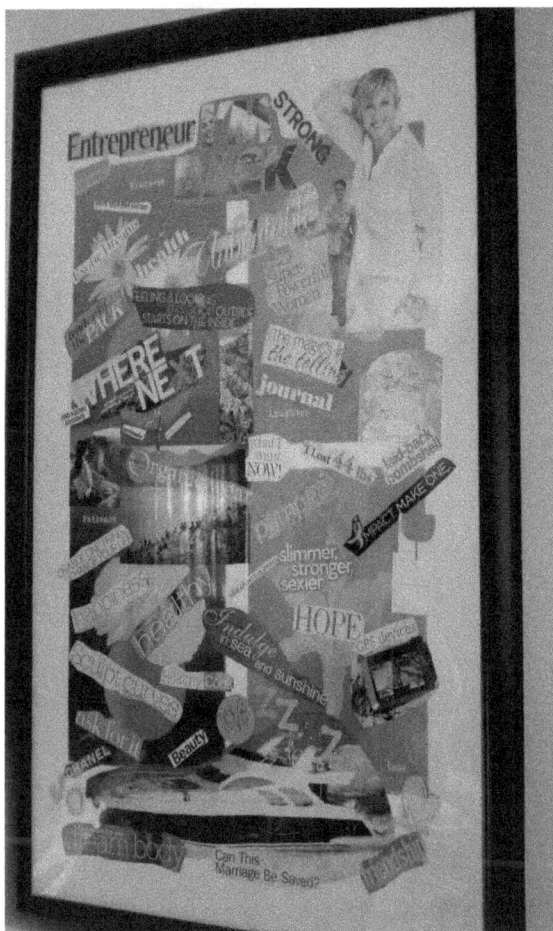

Reviewing both Vision Boards I have achieved almost everything on them – how cool is that! Some people make fun of Vision Boards however, I believe what you conceive can be achieved through action. They hang in my office today so I never forgot how far I have come and will never stop dreaming BIG.

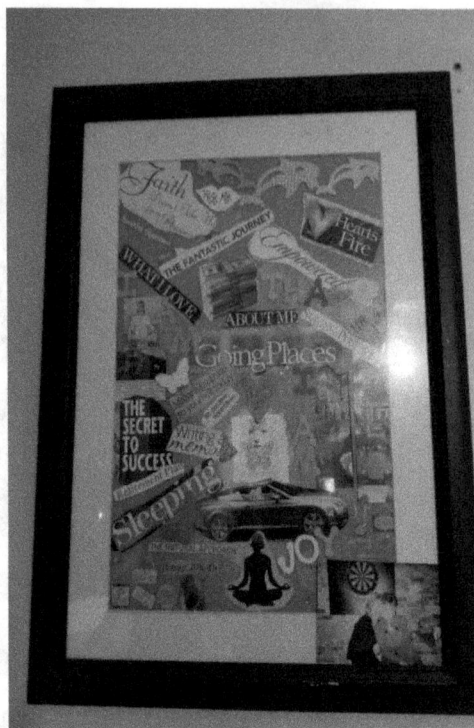

Becoming a Stress Management Coach opened my closed mind to believe that all things are possible.

NEGATIVE SELF-TALK

I stopped my negative self-talk using a rubber band. In 2004, I took an anger management course and the Instructor shared a technique using a rubber band. If this is an issue for you, put a thick rubber band around your wrist. Every time you have a negative thought about yourself or you become angry for no reason STOP right then and pull on the rubber band and let it go. It is quite painful so it forced me to stop negative self-talk in a few days. It also calmed me down when I got angry or impatient. I would snap it as hard as I could. It works real fast.

I hope you understand how important it is to have positive ENERGY flowing through you and around you. Life is so much grander with a positive MINDSET. Everything is energy and it has an actual frequency, hertz measurement. The human body is 100% energy. We can only attract people and situations to us that resonate at the same frequency.

Think of how important that statement truly is. If we run at a low frequency of negative thought patterns or attitude what usually comes to us but low energy and usually negative situations or results. When you raise your consciousness, think positive thoughts, still the mind, use visualization, it will raise your magnetic vibration. You will be amazed how quickly you can turn around any situation. It really is that easy!

Why do we make everything so difficult? I refuse to dwell on anything negative longer than one hour. I make it a personal challenge not to allow anyone or anything to shut my light off. I will not give my power away to any thought or person. You then become this manifesting machine....

Whatever you think about, you bring about. It really is that easy. Why must we beat ourselves up for the past? We cannot change the past, so do not let it define you. Forgive yourself and make the decision to push past the BS that does not serve us.

It is now time for you to take your power back! Time to be

first on your list! Time to get out of your own way!

I guarantee when you make these slight energy and mindset shifts, your life will change in lightning speed.

It has been an amazing journey to date. I have resonated the most loving friendships of like-minded individuals that have become my family. How does it get any better than that?

Don't think about what can happen in a month. Don't think about what can happen in a year. Just focus on the next 24 hours in front of you and do what you can to get closer to where you want to be.

CRAP YOUR EGO SAYS
Listen to your spirit!

YOUR EGO SAYS	YOUR SPIRIT SAYS
I am a **victim** of circumstances.	I create my **own** reality.
I live in scarcity. There is **never** enough.	I live in abundance. There is **always** enough.
I am **always** screwing up.	My path is sacred. I am **always** in the right place.
I need to **prove** my worth.	I **am** worthy.
I am in **competition** with the world.	I am in FLOW with the world.

kItt Depatie 3.16

It is time to forgive and forget all who have hurt you. No more should of, would of, could of mentality. It is time to be responsible for your life choices. So, say goodbye to what does not serve you. Forgive those from past hurts, however,

forgiveness of self, most importantly, because that is the only way we can move forward in life.

We all want happiness, love, joy, confidence, success, good health, and to be heart connected in our daily life. The question is, how do we train our minds so this becomes second-nature?

FLIP the switch for Mindset Shift

Define the single most destructive limiting belief you have about yourself, (resentment, fear, anger, self-criticism).

Write down in white space provided a few limiting beliefs keeping you stuck or frustrated. Example, "I cannot complete a task that is important to me."

_____

_____

_____

_____

_____

_____

_____

_____

Write down a few positive mindset shifts you would like to achieve. Example, I write down my goals. I take daily action for accountability and achievement. I keep myself motivated.

_____

_____

_____

_____

_____

_____

_____

Identify the circumstances that typically bring negative thoughts to the forefront. Example, my family makes fun of my goals on the refrigerator.

_____

_____

_____

_____

_____

_____

Another technique you can stop negative self-talk is once it happens just say "CANCEL CANCEL" out loud. This worked famously for me as well. When I said it out loud it would make me laugh and it would instantly shift my mindset with a smile. If you incorporate either one of these easy tools you can shift in an instant. The coolest part of the process is, when you are ready to change your thoughts and actions in these critical moments, you systematically weaken the impulse. Sometimes, the limiting belief is dissolved the first time this takes place, others can require more time and effort, so be patient with yourself.

Gratitude is important too. Before bed write down 5 things you are grateful for and NO repeats. Each day try to go deeper in your journaling. How did you honor and love yourself? How did you pay it forward? Did you assist someone in need? Did you smile and make someone's day, etc.

When you do this consistently, you can make this thought replacement permanent, like I have. By replacing negativity with a mindset shift, you will improve the course of your life.

Einstein said, "We cannot solve the issues we face at the same level of thinking that created them. To change the results we are getting, we must start to systematically change the way we think, act, and make our lives the result of our very best thinking."

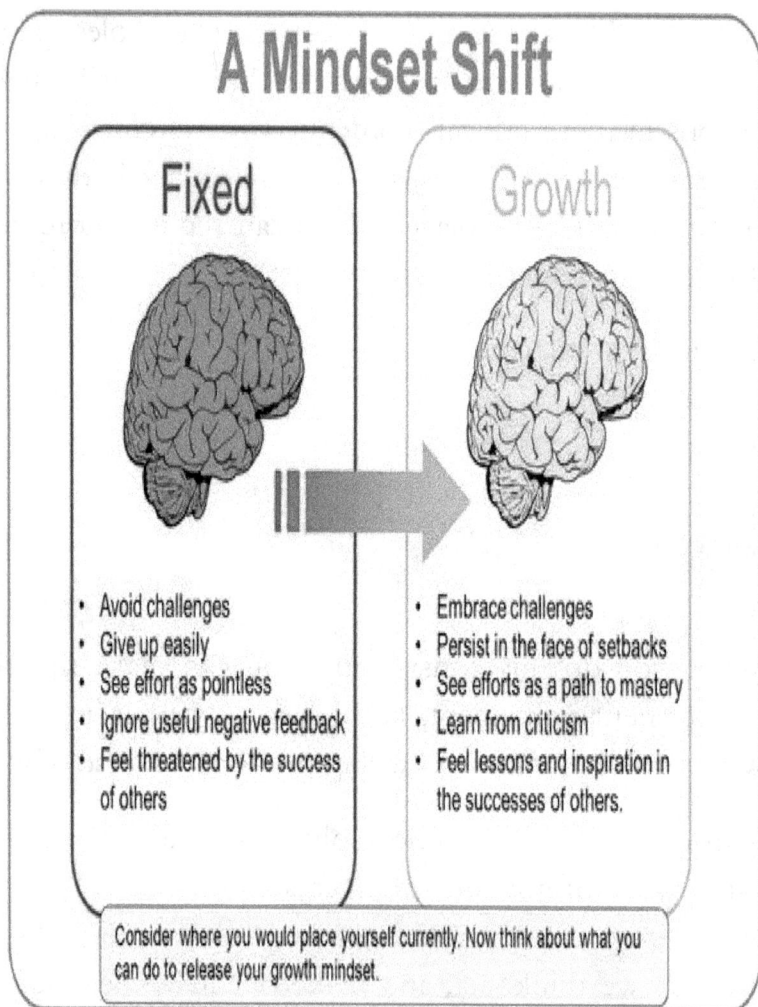

A Mindset Shift

Fixed

- Avoid challenges
- Give up easily
- See effort as pointless
- Ignore useful negative feedback
- Feel threatened by the success of others

Growth

- Embrace challenges
- Persist in the face of setbacks
- See efforts as a path to mastery
- Learn from criticism
- Feel lessons and inspiration in the successes of others.

Consider where you would place yourself currently. Now think about what you can do to release your growth mindset.

Create Positive Statements

I love and respect myself for who I am,
what I am, and what I bring to the world!

I am embracing change.

I am up for the challenge.

I am communicating effectively.

I am respectful of others.

I am honoring my feelings.

I am filled with passion and purpose.

I am emotionally available.

I am able to forgive those who have hurt me.

I am fearless.

I am open for all new possibilities.

I am happy and healthy.

Take some time to write your own I AM affirmations, notes, feelings, and action steps you would like to achieve. Begin with I AM...

_____

_____

3 EAT DIFFERENTLY

Why is it so important to listen to what your body tells you after eating? When I began to pay attention to how my body responded to my favorite foods, I found that pasta, pizza, bread, my daily go to, made my sinuses and throat close up, and felt bloated within 3o minutes. Hmm interesting!

When I began my health and wellness journey using my biofeedback machine, it blew me away all the food sensitivities I had. I did not realize how often my sinuses acted up and throat closed. I found this fascinating. I had to dive deeper and know more! I am Italian and have been raised on pasta, pizza, or bread almost every meal. When I felt down or depressed, I ate pasta with butter and all was well in my world! LOL – NOT! Those foods were my addiction and had no clue how toxic they were for my body.

I also began to consume grass fed protein, organic fruits, and veggies which to me tasted better, last longer, and my body was very satisfied. Some clients complain about the cost of organic foods. I question them, why is it important to spend money on alcohol or cigarettes, excess shopping, fast foods, expensive restaurants, but find it difficult to spend money on your health?   Isn't it important to invest in your health and wellbeing so the EMT's do not show up on your door step?

If not now when? If not this what? Are you not worth the investment to live a healthy and vibrant life?

Organic

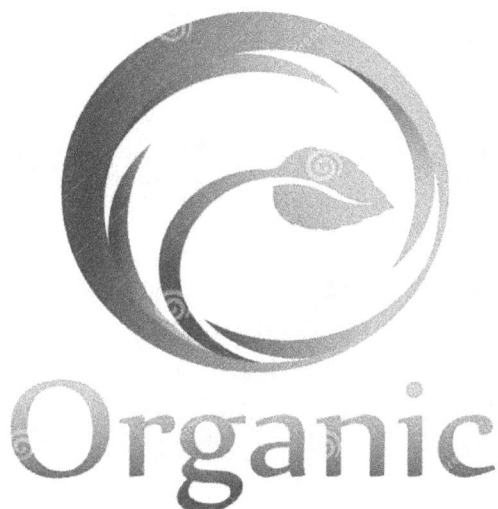

I decided years ago that my health was most important and after paying monthly responsibilities the rest is invested in my wellbeing.

I have tried over the last 30 years every diet, pill, drink, fat burner, extreme workouts, starving, fasting, Jenny Craig, you name it, yet, none of them kept the weight off until now.

I also battled weight up and down due to my thyroid being taken out when I was 17 years old. I was very active, ate the same foods my sister and brother did, and they did not put a pound on – it was so frustrating. I was called chubby, porky, big girl, and the list went on.

My body image has been an emotional roller coaster for most of my life. Especially, since I had a bean pole for a sister, Gina. I secretly wished I had her body growing up. That was then and now I love what I see in the mirror. Am I at my perfect weight? Almost! Do I work out 2 hours a day? NO.

I am 62 years young and it is 2019. What I do is love myself for where I am right now in this moment. I eat organic foods whenever possible. I walk the inter-coastal bridge with my accountability partner Bella girl, who never says NO 4 times a week when home. I hired Craig Long my trainer to assist me in building muscle and enhance my stamina and lost 11 pounds in 2 months. If I can do it so can you. My accountability partner Bella…love her so!

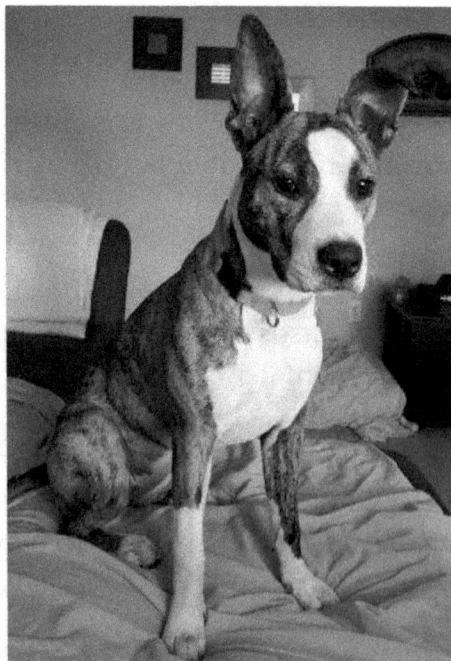

I recently hired a personal trainer, Craig Long, who loves to kick my butt 3 times a week! I am determined to rid my body of gluten and to reshape my body for the last time! Is it possible, yes, and with my coach no reason goal cannot be achieved.

My mindset is all about anti-aging and prevention. I see Dr. He, M.D., practicing acupuncture, 3 to 4 times a month to desensitize allergens. I take my eating plan seriously. I drink the best water possible. I keep bad foods out of my house so there are no temptations. I never go through a drive through and always have raw nuts, protein bars, and finger foods with me all the time which keeps me honest! It takes a bit of planning but my body loves me for it.

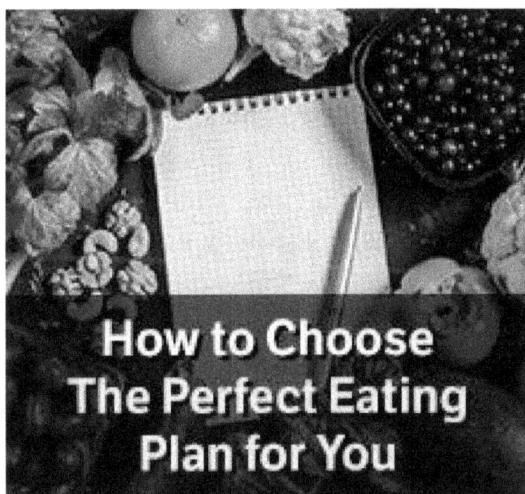

How to Choose The Perfect Eating Plan for You

When working with my clients we will discuss their current eating plan, review their food sensitivities with their biofeedback session, create a new eating plan for 90 days. I check in weekly and we discuss what changes they see with

eliminating said foods. Clients report their sleep improves, bloating gone, less fatigue, more energy, acid reflux gone, no more sugar cravings, etc. Your awareness is key.

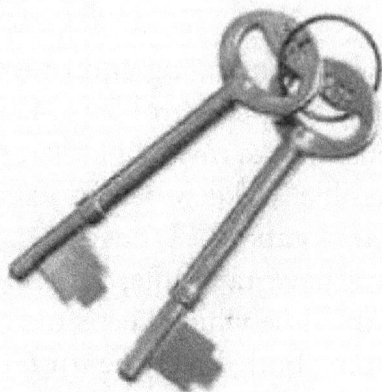

Most clients eat the same foods and this could be the reason why they become sensitive to them.

Client Case Study – Jenn came open to try a biofeedback session to figure out why she had so much abdominal pain. Jenn was treated by her Doctor and put on meds that did not work. She tried acupuncture with some relief but pain was still there.

We began her session and after the 3-minute scan I shared my findings. Her number one stressor was chicken and her second was grapes. Jenn confirmed that she only ate chicken and she drank a bottle of wine every night. I shared if she wanted the pain to go she had to remove those two items from her diet.

Jenn was in disbelief but said she would try it for one week. Guess what happened? Six months later, Jenn walked into the office and I did not recognize her. She lost 60 pounds in 6 months, changed her diet, used weight watchers, moved a little, and all her pain and cramping disappeared from her abdominal area. She was quite glad she did not let her Doctor give her a hysterectomy because they could not find anything wrong with her…

The stress in my brother's life also took a toll on his body. His acid reflux, alcoholism, diet, and negative emotions were the culprits that killed him. These stressors appeared in his biofeedback sessions but being diagnosed with Stage 4 cancer too late and not enough strength to fight. Do you know that cancer lives in an acidic body and thrives on sugar?

My friend Ursula was told she had 3 months to live and she said, "NO WAY not happening to me." The mind and will of our spirit is an amazing tool we have in our personal tool chest. However, some people do not believe in a holistic approach to wellness. Nor will they do the intense work to change their lifestyle habits. A holistic approach is a journey but for those that are up for the fight I am here to cheerlead you every step of the way!

It has been my mission and life's work to teach, preach, inspire, and motivate YOU how important it is to listen to what your body is telling you. Are you listening?

Unfortunately, Western medicine is trained on what pill to take and this will NEVER fix one thing, rather it is masking

the symptom. If you want to look, feel, and thrive well past 95, it is time to look reduce your stress and what you put in your mouth.

Keeping your stress at bay, move your body, eat right foods, hydration, detoxing, are a few easy techniques that will keep you on track which can potentially add 10 – 15 years to your life. Without your health, what is the point!

Are you eating foods that are fresh or in a box? Are you going through the drive-through or cooking your meals daily? Do you shop on the outside perimeter of the store or in the middle?

Awareness is key. At the end of the day are you really giving your body core nutrition?

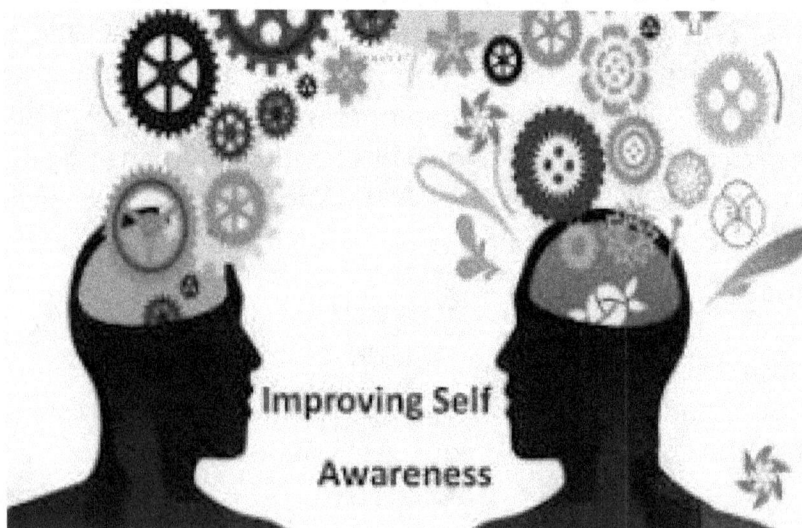

Improving Self Awareness

Do You Eat Franken foods?

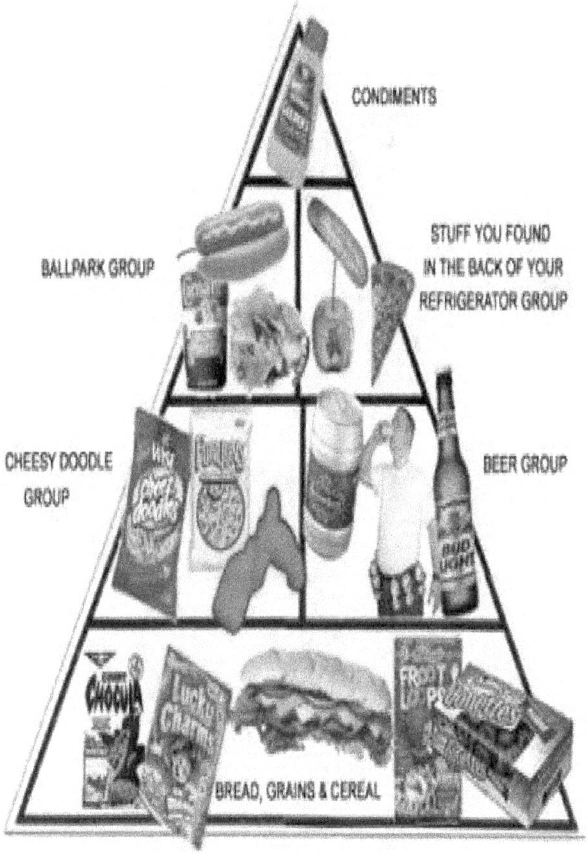

CONDIMENTS

STUFF YOU FOUND
IN THE BACK OF YOUR
REFRIGERATOR GROUP

BALLPARK GROUP

CHEESY DOODLE
GROUP

BEER GROUP

BREAD, GRAINS & CEREAL

Do you eat healthy foods?

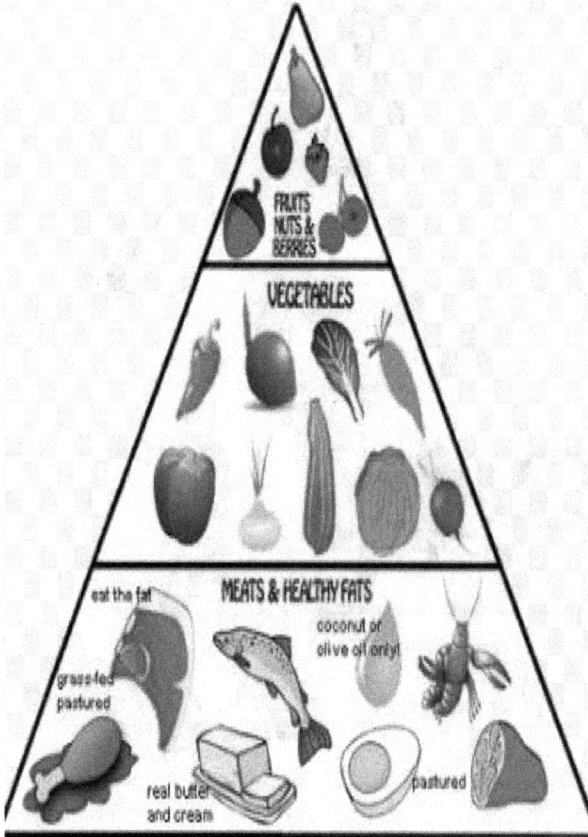

If you want to get your sexy back, feel better, reduce inflammation, gain energy, reduce joint pain and medication,

lower cholesterol, and so much more. Now is the time to listen to your what your body is saying. YOU are what you eat and drink it is really that simple.

It is time to EAT TO LIVE not live to eat! Shifting your mindset to fueling your body with core nutrition will make all the difference in the world!

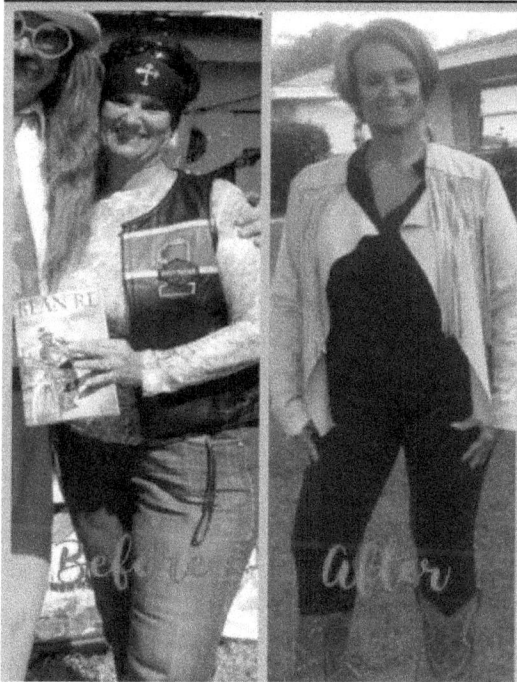

Doing sessions on myself taught me that I had many food sensitivities. My body was filled with inflammation due to eating the wrong foods that I loved. These three foods were my drug of choice pasta, bread, and pizza. I truly understand how difficult it is to get off drugs or alcohol. That was my drug of choice – carbs!

When I began to detox my body from GLUTEN it was awful. I truly was addicted. Carbs were not my friend and realized I ate over 1000 grams a day. I made the decision not to eat gluten for 30 days. I felt depressed, short-tempered, lack of energy, hard time sleeping, the cravings were crazy. GLUTEN is the silent killer for me! The importance of paying attention to what your body is telling you is critical.

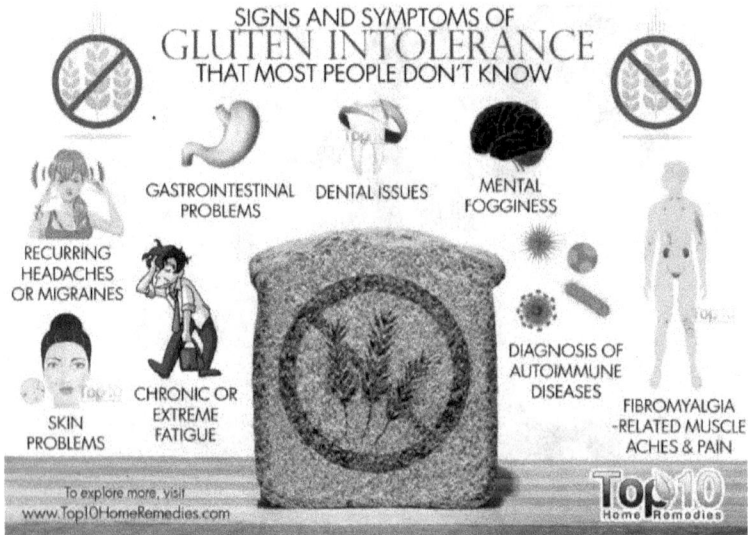

SIGNS AND SYMPTOMS OF
GLUTEN INTOLERANCE
THAT MOST PEOPLE DON'T KNOW

GASTROINTESTINAL PROBLEMS

DENTAL ISSUES

MENTAL FOGGINESS

RECURRING HEADACHES OR MIGRAINES

SKIN PROBLEMS

CHRONIC OR EXTREME FATIGUE

DIAGNOSIS OF AUTOIMMUNE DISEASES

FIBROMYALGIA -RELATED MUSCLE ACHES & PAIN

To explore more, visit www.Top10HomeRemedies.com

Top10 Home Remedies

Today all I need to do is clean my diet of toxic foods and the weight literally falls off. I used to live to eat because it was the only joy I found in my life. Once I began my health and wellness journey I stopped using foods to satisfy my depression because all it did was keep me depressed and addicted to carbs. I made a conscious choice to eat foods that keep me healthy and not just for taste.

4 MOVE Differently

You can make it fun and it is easy to add 30 minutes to your day to get the body moving. Stop being lazy or making excuses to get your work out in. If I can do it, so can you. Time to change your stinking thinking and get moving to the beat of a different drum.

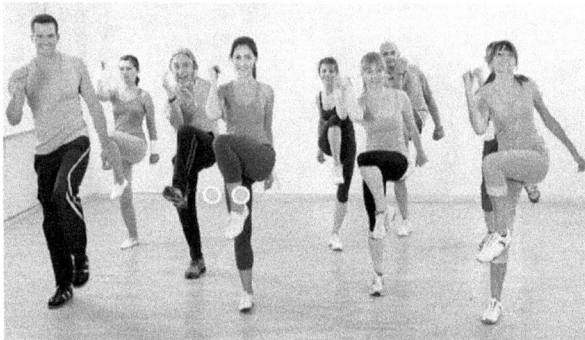

I travel often, so it is important for me to move my body. Taking Bella and walking the bridge is a magical way for me to begin my day. I get to witness sunrise, birds chirping, dolphins playing, and a quiet stillness that settles my soul for the day! It truly makes my spirit and soul sing and I get to collect my thoughts for the day. It is when creative nuggets come to me as well. Got to love it!

Another fun way to get moving is East and West Coast Swing. I joined a few dance clubs to get my body moving. I have so much fun being social and the cardio workout is fantastic. I smile from ear to ear and it brings me so much joy. My mom is 84 years young and is an East Coast Swing Dancer (Beach Boppers). I love to watch her in action. She had a knee replaced and stated if she could not dance any more she would rather die... Now if I could just get her to drink more water and eat healthier she would live well past 100 years!

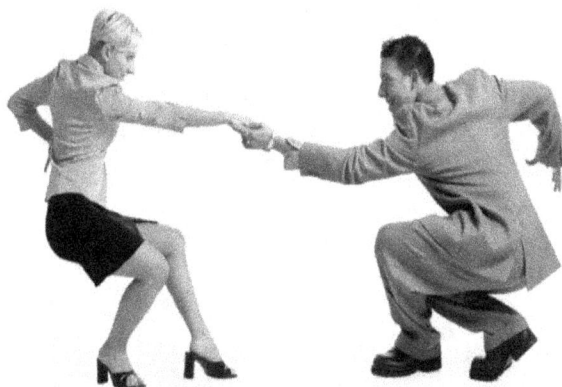

It is so easy to find on social media workouts that will fit into your busy schedule. It is time to love yourself enough to get moving. Stop the excuses and get your butt out of bed 30 minutes earlier - no more excuses. Nike's moto

JUST DO IT!

I also love Beach Body workouts, 21 Day Fix, to up my game while travelling. It is so easy to stay in shape if you incorporate the appropriate tools for your life style.

Another fun class I really enjoyed was aerial yoga. I highly suggest test driving a local YOGA class to reduce stress, great for relaxation, increase flexibility, sleep better, and it also enhances your breathing to name a few benefits.

Last year I was turned on to Aerial Yoga, thank you Tamela Staubs. I really enjoyed it and no stress on my joints. It is a must try. If you do not stay flexible through the aging process, all kinds of ailments begin to attack your body. Continued flexibility also plays an important role in allowing us to stay independent and not co-dependent on others.

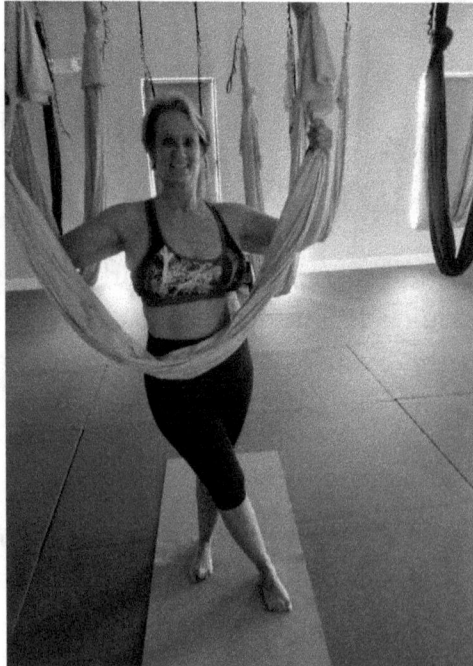

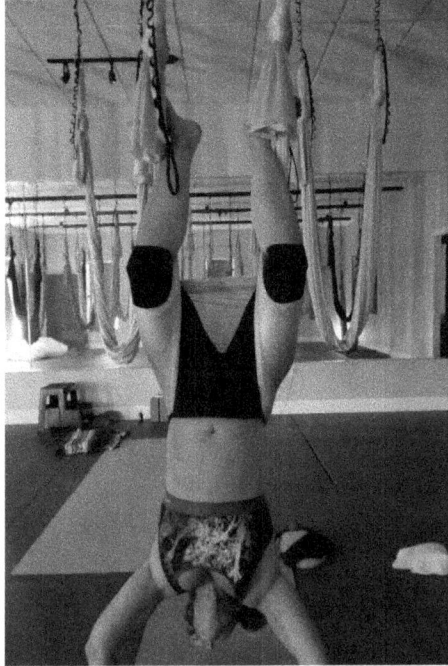

Posture & Circulation

When our muscles are limber, our bodies can relax. It's hard to keep good posture if our back, neck, chest and shoulder muscles are stiff and sore. Flexibility improves posture, which in turn helps to keep our spine and hips properly aligned and allows for better lung

capacity and breathing, which contributes to better circulation.

Enhanced Balance

When your muscles and joints are flexible, it's easier to keep your balance. A limber body can control its muscles and react quickly, keeping you upright even if you trip or slide. When muscles are tight, they don't adjust easily to sudden changes of position, and the accidental trip on the stairs could very well turn into a serious fall.

Preventing Injuries

Similarly, when you do experience a fall or other forceful impact, flexibility in the muscles and tendons surrounding your joints can determine whether or how bad of an injury you may incur. When muscles are stiff, your body won't move as easily to brace the hit. Tendons could strain, muscles could pull and fail to protect your bones and joints. Limber muscles can be the difference between a bruise and a busted hip.

A loss of flexibility doesn't have to happen as we get older. True, our joints, muscles and tendons do naturally lose elasticity with time, but we can work to get it back. Unlike strength and cardiovascular performance, flexibility doesn't have a cap when it comes to age, but we should work to

increase and maintain it before we experience an injury or start to feel stiff. These tips should help you get started.

Stretching

Experts suggest completing stretching exercises at least three times a week to keep your body flexible. Stretch your muscles to the point where they feel tight, but aren't causing you pain. If it hurts, ease up to where the pain stops and hold there. Stretching too far too fast can cause serious injuries.

Warm Up

Just like clay or taffy, muscles stretch better when they are warm. Consider doing stretching exercises after a few minutes of light cardio or after you take a shower.

Patience

If you know you're not as flexible as you once were, don't

expect your body to respond after just a few sessions of stretching. Your muscles take time to regain elasticity. Set realistic goals for yourself and take it slow.

Chi Kung and Tai Chi

If you'd rather incorporate flexibility training into strength and balance exercises, Chi Kung and Tai Chi are two great ways to combine your fitness goals. Both are slow-paced and adaptable for all ability level.

Good for the Mind

When you get moving it also has above-the-neck benefits too. For the past decade or so, scientists have pondered how exercising can boost brain function. Regardless of age or fitness level (yup, this includes everyone from mall-walkers to marathoners), studies show that making time for exercise provides some serious mental benefits.

Reduces Stress

Rough day at the office? Take a walk or head to the gym for a quick workout. One of the most common mental benefits of exercise is stress relief. Working up a sweat can help manage physical and mental stress. Exercise also increases concentrations of norepinephrine, a chemical that can moderate brain's response to stress. So, go ahead and get sweaty—working out can reduce stress and boost the body's ability to deal with existing mental tension. Win-win!

Boost Serotonin

Exercise releases endorphins, which create feelings of happiness and euphoria. Studies have shown that exercise can even alleviate symptoms among the clinically depressed. In some cases, exercise can be just as effective as antidepressant pills in treating depression. Don't worry if you're not exactly the gym rat type—getting a happy buzz from working out for just 30 minutes a few times a week can instantly boost overall mood.

Improve Self-Esteem & Confidence
Regardless of weight, size, gender, or age, exercise can quickly elevate a person's perception of his or her attractiveness, that is, self-worth.

Enjoy the Great Outdoors
For an extra boost of self-love, take that workout outside. Exercising in the great outdoors can increase self-esteem even more. Find an outdoor workout that fits your style, whether it's rock-climbing, hiking, renting a canoe, or just taking a jog in the park. Plus, all that Vitamin D acquired from soaking up the sun can lessen the likelihood of experiencing depressive symptoms. A little fresh air, sunshine, and movement can work wonders for self-confidence and happiness.

Prevent Cognitive Decline
It's unpleasant, but it's true—as we get older, our brains get a little hazy. As aging and degenerative diseases like Alzheimer's kill off brain cells, the brain shrinks, losing many important brain functions in the process. Exercise and a healthy diet can help shore up the brain against cognitive decline that begins after age 45. Working out, especially between age 25 and 45, boosts the chemicals in the brain that support and prevent degeneration of the hippocampus, an important part of the brain for memory and learning.

Alleviate Anxiety
Which is better at relieving anxiety—a warm bubble bath or

a 20-minute jog? You might be surprised at the answer. The warm and fuzzy chemicals that are released during and after exercise can help people with anxiety disorders calm down. Hopping on the treadmill for some moderate-to-high intensity aerobic exercise can reduce anxiety sensitivity.

Boost Brain Power

Various studies have shown that cardio-vascular exercise can create new brain cells and improve overall brain performance. Studies suggest that a tough workout increases levels of a brain-derived protein in the body, believed to help with decision making, higher thinking, and learning.

Sharpen Memory

Regular physical activity boosts memory and ability to learn new things. Getting sweaty increases production of cells in hippocampus responsible for memory and learning. For this reason, research has linked children's brain development with level of physical fitness.

Help Control Addiction

The brain releases dopamine, the "reward chemical" in response to any form of pleasure, be that exercise, sex, drugs, alcohol, or food. Unfortunately, some people become addicted to dopamine and dependent on the substances that produce it, like drugs or alcohol. On the bright side, exercise can help in addiction recovery. Short exercise sessions can also effectively distract drug or alcohol addicts, making them de-prioritize cravings in the short term. Alcohol abuse disrupts many body processes, including circadian rhythms. As a result, alcoholics find they can't fall asleep (or stay asleep) without drinking. Exercise can help reboot the body clock, helping people hit the hay at the right time.

Increase Relaxation

Ever hit the hay after a long run or weight session at the gym? For some, a moderate workout can be the equivalent of a sleeping pill, even for people with insomnia. Moving around five to six hours before bedtime raises the body's core temperature. When the body temp drops back to normal a few hours later, it signals the body that it's time to sleep.

Get More Accomplished

Feeling uninspired in the cubicle or office? The solution might be just a short walk or jog away. Research shows that workers who take time for exercise on a regular basis are more productive and have more energy than their more sedentary peers. While busy schedules can make it tough to squeeze in a gym session in the middle of the day, some experts believe that midday is the ideal time for a workout due to the body's circadian rhythms.

Tap into Creativity

Most people end a tough workout with a hot shower, but maybe we should be breaking out the colored pencils instead. A heart-pumping gym session can boost creativity for up to two hours afterwards. Supercharge post-workout inspiration by exercising outdoors and interacting with nature. Next time you need a burst of creative thinking, hit the trails for a long walk or run to refresh the body and the brain at the same time.

Accountability Partners

Whether it's a pick-up game of golf, a group class at the gym, or just a run/walk with a friend, exercise rarely happens in a bubble. Studies show that most people perform better on aerobic tests when paired up with a workout buddy. Even fitness beginners can inspire each other to push harder during a workout, so find a fitness buddy and get moving.

5 THINK Differently

You must think differently to change the course of your life. The definition of INSANITY is doing the same thing over and over again and expecting a different result. Let's stop the INSANITY...

Change Negative Thoughts to Positive

One of the most important things to do when changing your attitude is to stop thinking negative thoughts. We all have negative thoughts, but it is those of us who linger on them that will struggle to overcome them. The more you listen to those negative voices in your head, the more real they become. One thing to remember though is that they are only thoughts, not facts and you can change your reaction to them.

It's easy enough to tell someone to stay positive when they're feeling down. But how does a person alter the way they think? Human brains are trained to automatically go into defense mode when something goes wrong - this is the flight or fight mode we hear all so often. To change our reaction to negativity, we need to learn to differentiate real threats from imagined ones. Each time you have a negative thought write it down and ask yourself why. Is it as bad as you think it is? Chances are...it's not. Anytime you feel a negative thought creeping into your head try replacing it with something that makes you smile or get out that rubber band! Becoming a more positive person will not only improve your health but improve your career and personal life too!

Positive Thinking It's Contagious
Like a yawn, if someone sees you coming into the room with a spring in your step and a smile on your face it will rub off on them.

It helps you to solve problems
If you are already thinking in a positive way when you come across a problem, then you will find it easier to solve.

Improves performance
If you're in a good mood you will be more creative, more conscious in the moment, and more energetic than if you're feeling low.

Improves Health
It's well documented that positive thinking improves your health. If you're healthy and happy in your work, then you will be able to achieve anything you set your mind to do.

Improves Relationships
If you're one of those people that walks into a room and instantly brightens it up, people will be drawn to you and not the person hiding in the corner that never smiles!

If you have been struggling to achieve your targets, think about what you can do to improve and don't dwell too much on what went wrong. Positive thinking breeds success, and, if you incorporate this into your daily life, you'll smash those targets and achieve everything you set your mind to!

How Do You Handle Stress?
Stress affects people in all different ways – or at least, different people respond to it very differently. For some, it

rolls off quickly, and they rebound in a reasonable amount of time. For others, it "sticks" and it takes much longer to recover, if ever. This is because people's mental "resilience" varies enormously, which itself is based on both genes and environment. For people who do not cope well with stress, it may be that they've never been particularly good at it - or it could be that they were once good, but the losses and blows of life have worn away their resilience over time. Luckily, it's possible to build that skill back up.

We all experience terrible loss and hurdles at some point in our lives; the death of a loved one, a divorce or painful breakup, being fired from a job, suffering from an illness, or any number of life events that can be overwhelming and terrifying to confront.

Some people can bounce back quicker than others. People that struggle longer, with higher incidences of depression, anxiety, and long-term effects of stress that take a toll on their lives. The good news is that resilience is a learned technique and getting to the root cause of it is the key to understanding and then changing the pattern.

Stretch Your Mental Muscle

People often have a go-to coping method, which may or may not be effective in every life event. The thing that resilient people know is that different challenges require different strategies. So, learning how to pick and choose your response in any given situation is key. Flexibility means you

approach any hurdle with a variety of strategies. Sometimes you need to lean on others and get emotional support. Other times you need to give yourself space to heal or grieve or let things cool off. Some situations need swift and strong action to advocate for yourself or confront a situation head on. You can practice this by noticing your go-to method of coping, and then deliberately taking a step back.

Most people know at least intellectually that first reactions aren't always the best ones—it usually takes some space to fully digest the situation before you can settle on the best response. Make sure you give yourself adequate time to do this, so that you can come up with the best method, rather than just using the first one that comes to mind.

Focus on Awareness of Triggers

When something bad happens that is your fault, try to use it to learn what you could have done better, rather than berate yourself.

During tough times or a difficult moment, you have a fundamental choice to respond with your old-patterns (e.g., defend, protect, attack, hide) or to open yourself to learning from the lesson that appears. I believe the UNIVERSE continues to bring our life lessons to us again and again until we learn from it, react differently, then it no longer appears, and we can move forward. I shared my life lesson in the first chapter. It truly took me until my mid-40s to figure out this game called life. I now move forward through any situation with ease and grace knowing that it is in divine order. The same will happen for you but awareness is key.

Become Physically Tougher

Getting in physical shape can do volumes for your mental well-being, resilience included. Part of being resilient is that you feel, at least to some degree, that you have control over your response to a situation (even if not the situation itself), and that you can problem-solve whatever challenges come up. When you're out of shape physically, it can feel like you're not in control of your body, let alone the stressors in your life. So just the act of getting in shape can be extremely empowering.

Keep Your Tank Energetically Full

This can be tough because life can be incredibly exhausting, especially if you're dealing with a series of stressors, and it's very easy to put your other commitments ahead of yourself. Work, spouse, kids, family all tend to get the better part of your energy. However, if you do not take care of yourself daily and replenish your mental energy, you will not be able to deal with stress that gets in your way.

It's difficult to be resilient to personal and professional challenges if you are already drained. If you don't get the sleep your body needs, eat good food, get fresh air and exercise, and some quiet time to reflect your response to a negative situation will not be favorable and then you come from fight or flight response.

Resilient people know that you need to keep a little fuel in the tank always. They know this isn't being selfish or lazy, but is a strong choice to put yourself in the best physical and emotional state for when inevitable challenges arise.

This book is all about potentially adding 10 – 15 years to your life. Prevention and anti-aging techniques start with thinking differently. If you are not feeling your best do not wait until an EMT shows up at your house or office to make a shift, it just may be too late.

How Do You Perceive Yourself?

This can be hard to do, since it can feel weird to write about yourself. Studies show that it's extremely good for mental health. Those who see themselves in a positive light tend to be more positive and resilient to stress than others that are more self-effacing. They even recover from tragedy and loss more quickly....... you can increase your resilience by boosting your ego in direct ways.

This could be fun to do as a family. Have everyone send you a quick video of how they perceive you. You will be surprised by what you learn, and it opens the door to honest communication in the family too.

A Highly Sensitive Person

Sensitive people often seem to have a harder time bouncing back from stressors, which
makes sense, since the impact of certain events tend to be magnified for them. But there's good news for the highly sensitive among us: They also tend to be very good learners when it comes to coping strategies. So, they may ultimately have a leg up with resilience, once they learn exactly how to deal with it.

6 INFLAMMATION

Inflammation is the root of all evil from what I have studied over the years! Did you know that most diseases are caused by inflammation in the body?

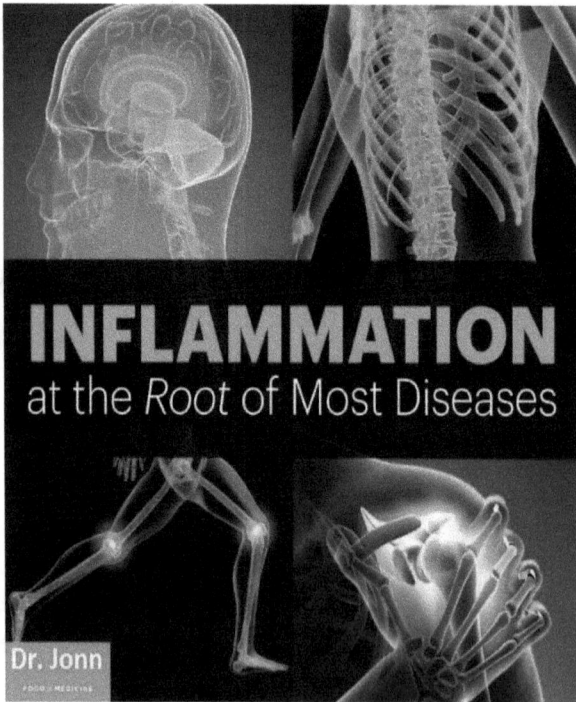

INFLAMMATION
at the *Root* of Most Diseases

Dr. Jonn

Article-Dr. David Marquis, DC, DACBN

"A wide array of health problems, including not limited to chronic pain, obesity, ADD/ADHD, neuropathy, diabetes, heart disease, stroke, migraines, thyroid issues, dental issues, and cancer are all rooted in inflammation, which must be properly addressed if you wish to be healed."

"The majority of inflammatory diseases start in the gut with an autoimmune reaction which progresses into systemic inflammation. When the intestinal lining is repeatedly damaged due to reoccurring leaky guy syndrome, damaged cells microvilli become unable to do their job properly. They become unable to process and utilize nutrients and enzymes that are vital to proper digestion. As more exposure occurs, your body initiates an attack on these foreign invaders. It responds with inflammation, allergic reactions, and other symptoms we relate to as a variety of diseases."

Inflammation Triggers/Symptoms of Disease

Allergies	Alzheimer's
Anemia	Asthma
Autism	Arthritis
Carpal Tunnel	Celiac
Chron's	Eczema
Congestive Heart Failure	
Fibromyalgia	Fibrosis
Gall Bladder Disease	Acid Reflux
Thyroiditis	Heart Attacks
Kidney Failure	Lupus
MS	Pancreatitis
Psoriasis	Stroke
Rheumatoid Arthritis	Scleroderma

"The presence of inflammation is what makes most disease perceptible to an individual. It can and often does occur for years before it exists at levels sufficient to be apparent or clinically significant. How long it has been smoldering really determines the degree of severity of a disease and often the prognosis assuming the inflammation can be controlled."

There are several ways to reduce inflammation from the body and I found a product that has 32 anti-inflammatories in it which caused me to drop 16" and 22 pounds in 6 weeks. I was blown away by my results, and had no clue I was filled with inflammation due to gluten intolerances. When something works and only costs $3.50 a day it was a no brainer for me!

Most nutritionists, trainers, athletes, and body builders recommend eating 4 to 6 small meals per day I finally did it and lost 8 lbs. in 3 weeks. It did work for me and had to plan my meals. However, some clients find it to be too much work!

My Mentor, Joel Bauer, and sister, Brenda, found their meal plan which is intermitted fasting. This allows you to eat bigger meals with less food prep. Here is some info to test drive and see if it works for you.

Intermittent Fasting (I.F.).
It's a type of eating that restricts food intake to a short time period each day. Usually a 4 to 8-hour window. Studies show that you only need about 16 hours of being in a fasted state to reap the largest benefit of IF or autophagy.

Autophagy is your body's natural "cell-cleaning" process. Basically, it removes dead and damaged tissue, and replaces it with new healthy tissue. For pain and inflammation, this is a powerful weapon. By activating your body's natural autophagy process, you suppress inflammation. You also slow down the aging process and boost natural energy hormones.

So, what does 16 hours of fasting look like? If you have dinner at 7pm then you don't eat again until 11am the following day... that's a 16 hour fast. You eat 2 to 3 small meals from 11 – 7 pm.

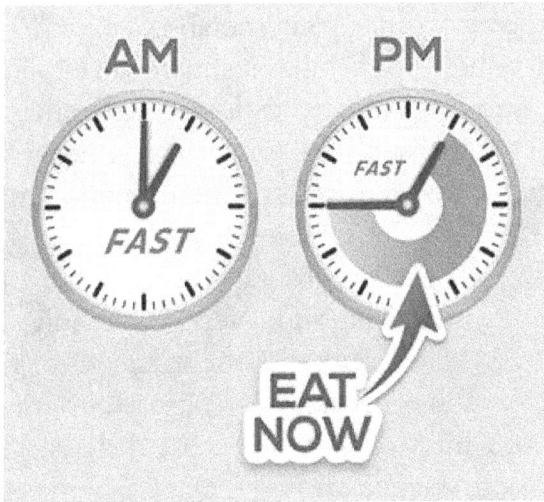

This example demonstrates a 16 hour fast from 9 p.m. until 1 p.m. the following day. Basically, skipping breakfast and eating the first meal of the day at lunch-time. Which means all you really need to do is skip breakfast to activate autophagy and reap the benefits of fasting. You may be less hungry on this regimen, like Brenda and Joel.

A study published in the American Journal of Physiology showed that after a 48-hour fast, **patients burned 3.6% more calories!** Even after 2 full days without food, these people didn't experience a drop in metabolic output. Instead, they experienced an uptick in calorie burning power. So, you'll be just fine going for a few hours without food. Your metabolism won't come to a screeching halt, and you won't lose all your muscle mass.

ANTI-INFLAMMATORY DIET

Eat *more* fat. Not only is fat an essential macronutrient for optimal human health. There are specific types of fat that boost brainpower, stoke your metabolism, and support fat-burning hormones. Studies have shown that following a low carb diet is an effective way to lower inflammation. This is absolutely true, I lost 4" on each thigh when taking gluten out of my diet which reduced the inflammation in my body.

Another suggestion is replacing certain high-carbohydrate foods with healthier, high-fat versions. Sadly, most diets suggest that you stay away from these fats. Not only are you missing out on some of the most powerful Super Foods on the planet, you miss out on the most delicious entrees and desserts! Good science shows that certain types of fat are heart-healthy, fat-loss friendly. They also help you build strong, pain-free joints.

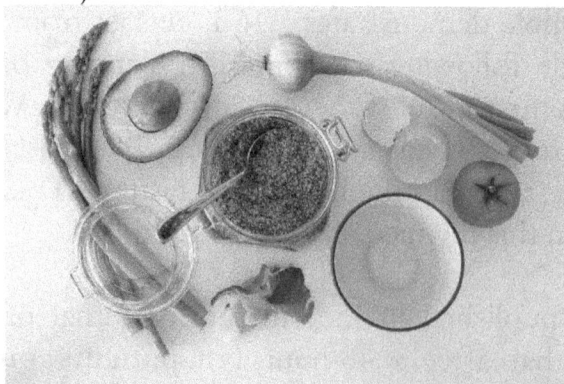

Adding specific high-fat foods to your diet helps regulate appetite hormones and inflammation levels.

It's vital that you consume adequate levels of these important types of fat to maintain hormonal health and a slim waistline. Your "low fat" diet could be why you aren't able to lose those last few pounds. I'll show you how to incorporate these fats into your daily routine in just a moment.

Remember this?

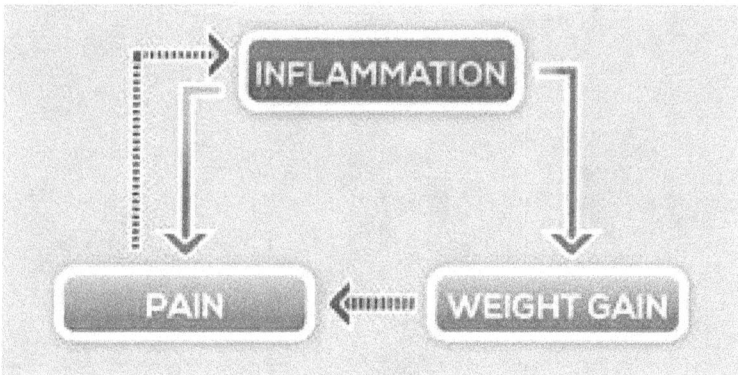

This is the cycle that you need to **break** to look, feel, and live potentially 10 – 15 years longer by reducing inflammation in the body. It's not your metabolism that needs fixed. It's not better drugs or more anti-inflammatory pills. It is now time to break the inflammation, weight gain, and pain cycle now.

It is time to break the cycle. It can be easy, it does work, and you can do it... I am here to support you each step of the way. Isn't it time to get your sexy back, feel great, more energy, sleep better, and be the best version of you?

Do your due diligence, find what works for you, and go to

your next family or High School reunion looking 10 to 15 years younger than your class. Now that is something to celebrate. Let's go…

7 DETOXIFICATION

Our bodies can become overwhelmed due to the volume of toxins exposed in its environment by way of water (fluoride and other chemicals), air (chemical trails, pollution and other toxins), food (chemicals, pesticides, preservatives, genetically modified ingredients etc.), pharmaceuticals and other drugs.

True healing requires a detoxification of both the mind and the body. Below are 10 ways you can help your body detoxify naturally so it can flush out some of the everyday toxins to which it's exposed:

- Start the day with a glass of spring organic lemon water, ginger root, and some honey if you would like. This will get things flowing in the morning and will begin your day being alkaline.

- Also, you can add a couple of tablespoons of apple cider vinegar to a glass of spring water. Hippocrates treated his patients with apple cider vinegar. He found it was a powerful cleansing and healing elixir, a naturally occurring antibiotic and antiseptic that fights germs and bacteria, for a healthier, stronger, and longer life.

- You must drink plenty of water throughout the day to continue flushing out the toxins.

- Drink a freshly made vegetable juice daily. Include lots of greens such as kale, spinach and cilantro. I love to start my day with a juice made with apples, carrot, lemon, ginger, turmeric, beetroot, kale and cilantro. When the seasons change, some of my ingredients will also change.

- Eliminate toxic oils from your diet. Like vegetable oil, peanut oil, sunflower oil, cotton seed oil and canola oil. Substitute with good oils, such as extra-virgin olive oil, coconut oil, avocado oil, hemp oil and flaxseed oil. Hemp oil, for example, is a great source of omega 3s, 6s, 9s.

- Drink green tea and herbal teas such as dandelion, nettles, etc. These teas help the body detoxify and clear out toxins.

- Eat more raw fruits, herbs and vegetables. Fruit, vegetables and herbs contain enzymes that aid digestion and improve nutrient absorption.

- Eliminate white sugar intake a silent killer for sure. Also avoid substitutes that contain toxic artificial sweeteners, and opt for natural versions such as stevia, honey, coconut sugar, date sugar, molasses, or maple syrup.

- Eliminate white flour and white breads (gluten free options). White flour is like adding glue in the body, and it overworks the digestive system. It can cause digestive disorders, and it can make it difficult to have normal bowel movements.

  Substitute white flour with other flours such as spelt flour, kamut flour, quinoa flour, brown rice flour, buckwheat flour or cornmeal. Switch from white bread to whole grain bread.

- Take a probiotic supplement. You can also eat foods that contain live cultures, such as cultured vegetables, Greek yogurt, or kefir. The beneficial bacteria kill harmful bacteria and yeasts and help to heal the lining of the intestines.

- Eat more legumes and less meat, fish and poultry. Legumes are a great source of protein and the fiber in beans helps keep the bowels eliminating properly.

- Breathe deeply, walk, smile, laugh, be happy and remove toxic people out of your life.

Find the positive and move your body every day. This will assist in reducing stress and the toxic chemicals that invade our body.

8 SUPRESSION

Appetite is generally a sign of good health; however, there are times when your appetite might run out of control and cause you to eat more than you should or want to. As a result, it puts you at risk for gaining unwanted weight and developing serious diseases. At times such as these you want to suppress your appetite naturally to stay fit and healthy.

Starving yourself is not the answer as that will only lead to binge eating. But turning to natural foods to suppress your appetite naturally will help to reduce appetite while supplying the body with much needed nutrition.

The difference between natural and unnatural foods is that natural foods are compatible with the human body, whereas unnatural foods are not. Natural foods are cleansing to the body and will eliminate any impurities in the bloodstream that cause overeating. Unnatural foods, on the other hand, are toxic to the body because the body is unable to process them efficiently, if at all. Over time they accumulate in the body causing weight gain and other diseases.

The following is a short list of natural foods that you can add to your daily diet to bring a healthy balance to your appetite.

Some of them might sound strange in the sense that they can help with weight loss, but tests show that they do help when added into a daily diet.

Wheatgrass

Wheatgrass is probably the best remedy to reduce your appetite. It is loaded with vitamins and minerals that help to satisfy your cravings. In addition, it is very cleansing and immediately begins to remove residues of unhealthy and fattening foods from the bloodstream. Naturally you crave what is in the bloodstream, and once the substances from unhealthy foods are removed, your cravings for them are removed as well. After that it becomes a mind-over-matter issue.

Fresh Fruit and Vegetable Juices

Fresh fruit and vegetable juices are also loaded with tons of vitamins and minerals that will naturally suppress your appetite. At first, these juices might increase appetite. This occurs when the body is toxic and malnourished. Once those toxins are removed, the juice is so filling that it can be taken as a substitute for a snack or even replace a meal.

Natural Appetite Suppressants

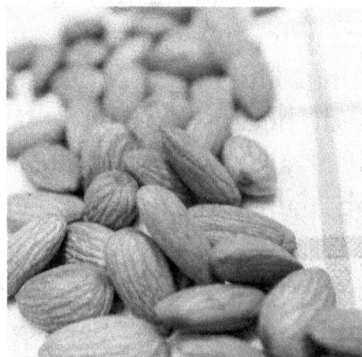

Just a handful of **almonds** is a rich source of antioxidants, vitamin E, and magnesium. Almonds have also been shown to increase feelings of fullness in people and help with weight management.

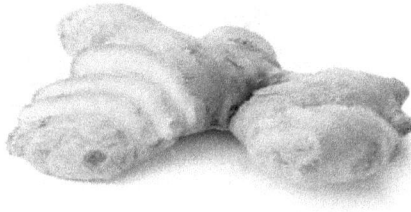

For centuries, many cultures have used **ginger** root for its amazing digestive powers. Whether it's in a smoothie or in an Indian dish ginger works as a stimulant that energizes the body and improves digestion, thereby making you less hungry.

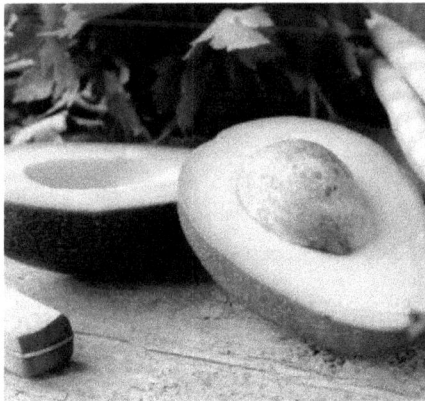

Full of fiber and heart-healthy mono-saturated fat, **avocados** suppress appetite when eaten in moderation. In fact, the fats in these little guys send signals to your brain that tell your stomach that it's full.

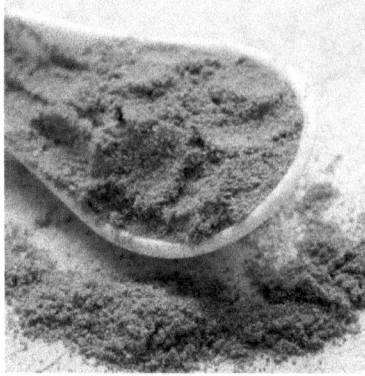

Time to get spicy! According to recent research just half a teaspoon of **cayenne pepper** can boost metabolism and cause the body to burn an extra 10 calories on its own. Adding cayenne pepper cuts an average of 60 calories from their next meal.

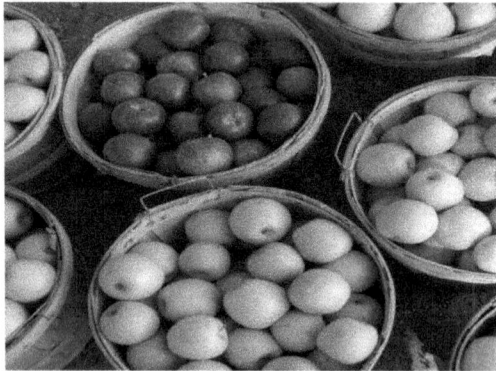

Apples of all varieties and types help suppress hunger. First, apples are filled with soluble fiber and pectin, which help you feel full. Apples also regulate your glucose and boost your energy level. Finally, apples require lots of chewing time, which helps slow you down and gives your body more time to realize that you're no longer hungry. Plus, they just taste good.

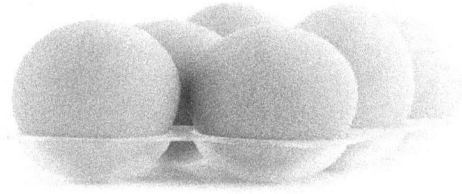

Studies have shown that eating an **egg** or two for breakfast can help dieters feel full over 24 hours than if they eat a bagel with the same number of calories.

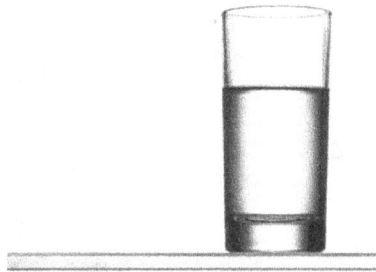

Could taming your appetite be as easy as drinking an extra glass or two of **water**? Science says yes! In one August 2010 study, people who drank two glasses of water before a meal ate between 75 and 90 fewer calories at the meal than those who didn't drink water.

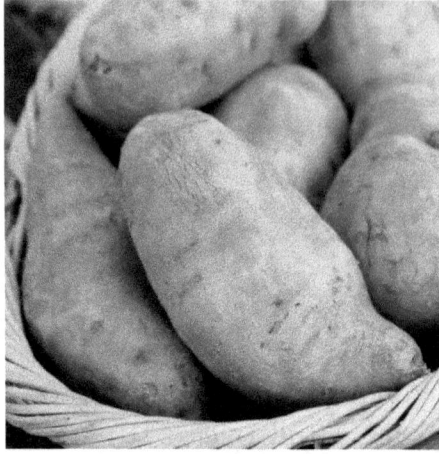

According to food scientists, **sweet potatoes** contain a special type of starch that resists digestive enzymes, making them stay in your stomach longer and therefore keep you full. Plus, they're full of vitamin A and vitamin C!

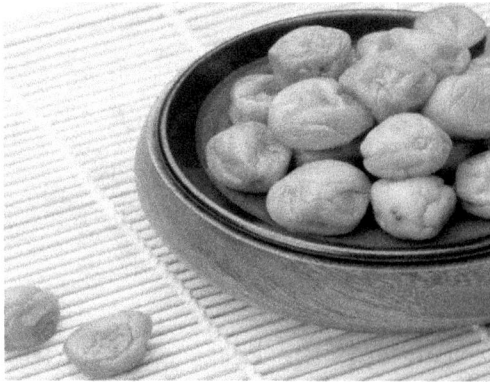

Have a sweet craving you just can't shake? Sometimes the best thing to do is to shock it with something sour. **Umeboshi plums** are basically pickled plums and can be fantastic for squashing sugar cravings. Find them at your local specialty store or Asian grocer.

A hot, **broth-based vegetable soup** can fill you up in a hurry and take the edge off your hunger with minimal calories. Try having a cup before your next meal or simply have a big bowl as your main course!

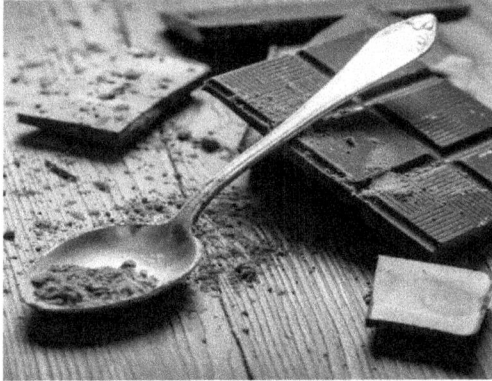

My favorite treat, **dark chocolate**, slowly savor a piece or two of dark chocolate with at least 70 percent cocoa the next time you crave it. Just a little dark chocolate helps to lower your cravings because the bitter taste signals the body to decrease your appetite. Not to mention that the steric acid in dark chocolate helps slow digestion to help you feel fuller longer.

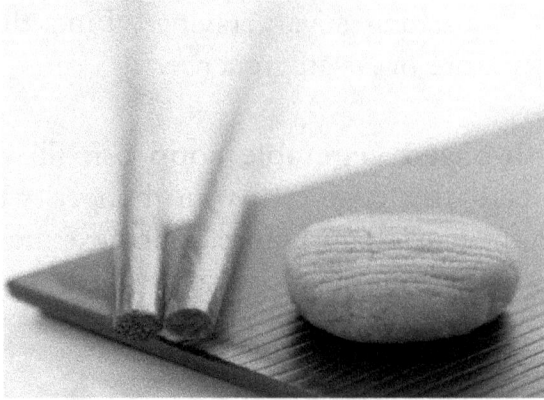

Ever notice how when you eat sushi it doesn't seem to take as much food to fill you up? Well, part of that is because of the healthy fish in sushi, but the other part is due to that spicy green stuff: wasabi! The spiciness in wasabi suppresses appetite and is a natural anti-inflammatory.

If you're not a coffee drinker and get sick of water easily, try sipping on a cup of hot green tea. **Green tea** can help you to stop mindlessly snacking, and nutritionists say that the catechins in green tea help to inhibit the movement of glucose into fat cells, which slows the rise of blood sugar and prevents high insulin and subsequent fat storage. And when your blood sugar is more stable so is your hunger!

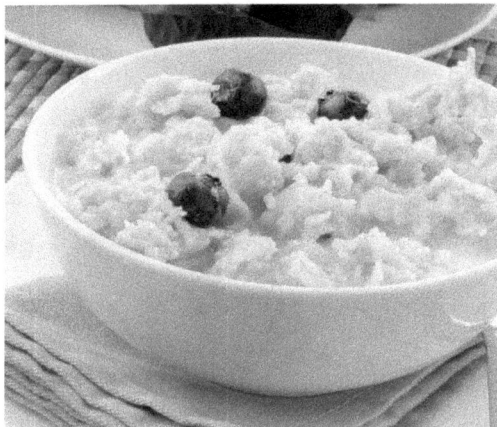

While high in carbs, the type of carbs in **oatmeal** are slow-digesting and keep you feeling full for hours after breakfast. Why? Because they suppress the hunger hormone ghrelin. In fact, oatmeal is low on the glycemic index—just be sure to choose steel cut oats to get the most benefit!

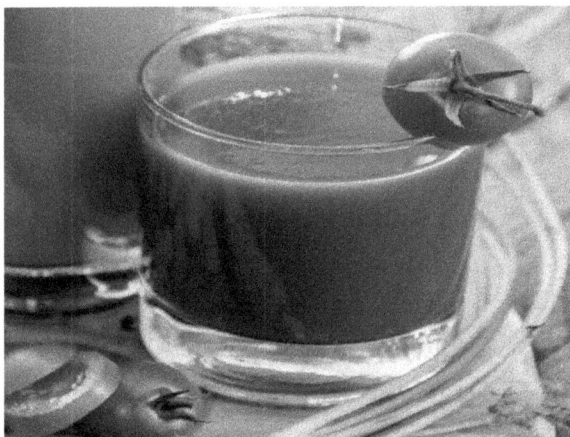

Veggie juice has been shown to fill you up. When you drink vegetable juice before a meal, you end up eating 135 fewer calories. Drink the low-sodium varieties, which are less likely to make you bloat.

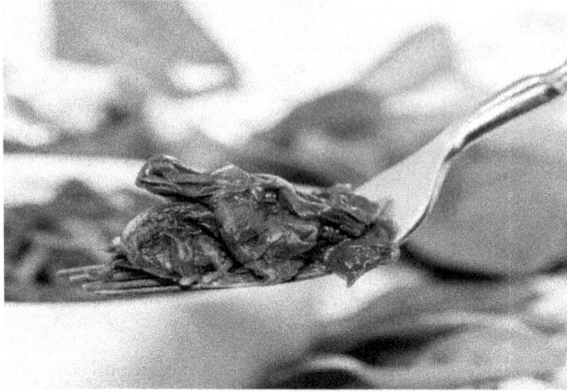

A highly nutritious food that will fill you up for hours, you can't **beat green leafy vegetables**. From kale to spinach to Swiss chard, these fibrous greens (eaten raw or gently sautéed with a little olive oil) are delicious and will keep hunger at bay.

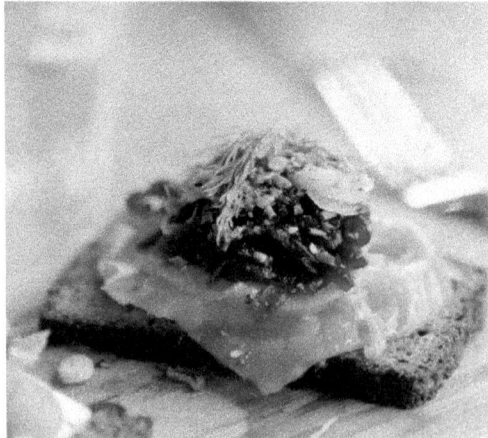

Salmon is high in Omega 3 fatty acids; your body increases the amount of the hormone leptin in your system. Leptin is known for suppressing hunger. Don't like salmon? Try tuna and herring, which are also high in omega-3s!

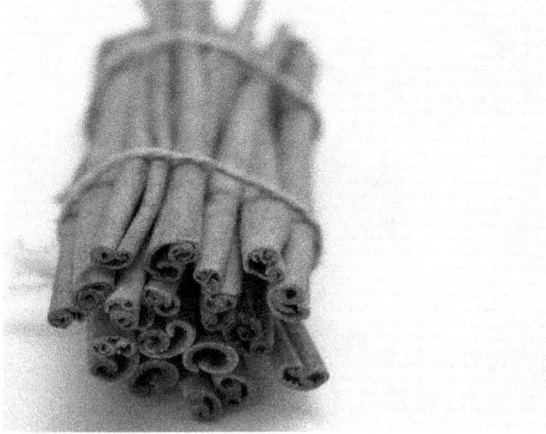

Next time you have cereal, oatmeal, fruit, or even coffee, sprinkle some cinnamon on it. Cinnamon, like other ground spices such as cloves and ginger, helps lower your blood sugar levels, which—you guessed it—helps to control your appetite!

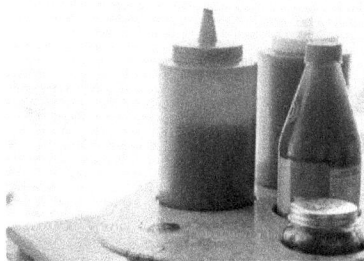

When it comes to hot sauce and appetite suppression, the hotter you can go the better. So, get your favorite hot sauces or some **Tabasco** and sprinkle some heat on your burrito, scrambled eggs, or even soup! The spiciness keeps you from overeating and helps you to stay full longer!

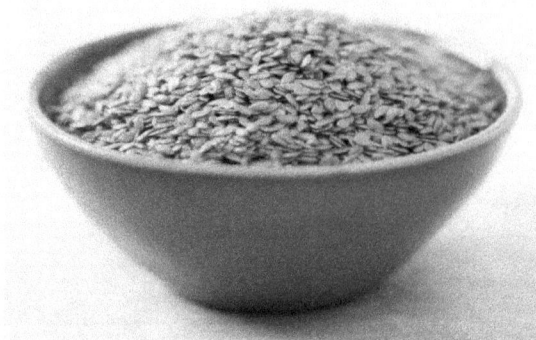

With a nutritional mix of soluble fiber and essential fatty acids, **flax seeds** are the perfect addition to your yogurt, smoothie, or salad. In fact, ground or whole, flax seeds help you to stay satiated and fueled!

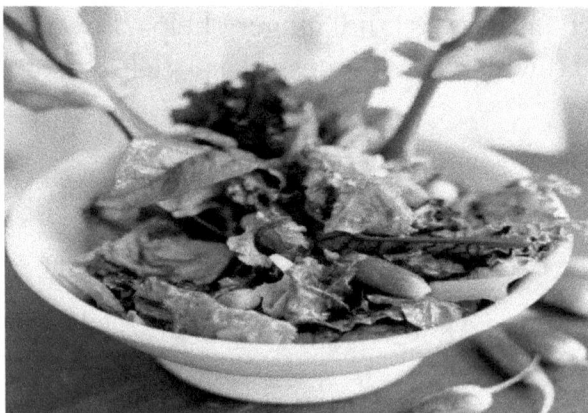

Eat a small salad before you sit down for a meal. Just a cup or two of veggies is all it takes to signal to your brain that you're getting calories and nutrition. It takes about 20 minutes for your stomach to feel full it is a perfect way to get a head-start, so you don't over eat.

9 THYROID

At the age of 17 I had a golf ball size tumor in my throat area and was diagnosed with a Goiter and Hashimoto's Disease. I went the follow week for surgery and they removed 90% of my thyroid. I have been on medication ever since and I am now 62 years old. I really had no clue about what that meant but they did the surgery and went back to high school to graduate. Here are some of the symptoms I had:

- Goiter, Enlargement of thyroid gland

- Fatigue

- Weight Gain

- Weakness

- High Cholesterol

- Depression – High Low Mood Swings

- Rapid Heart Beat

- Appetite Fluctuations

It is so important to find the right Thyroid Endocrinologist, Functional Medicine Professional, or Oriental Doctor that will listen to you. I also see many clients that have TSH, T3, or T4 issues but their Doctor will tell them their blood work fits in the normal range. It is not normal to feel the way you feel please seek out additional advice.

Rich Food Sources of Iodine

It is very important to include high amounts of iodine rich foods in your diet as the body cannot synthesize this mineral. The amount of iodine found in food sources is small. The quantity of iodine depends on environmental factors like use of fertilizers and soil concentration. Here is a list of the best iodine rich foods.

Sea Vegetables

Sea vegetables contain excellent sources of iodine. Kelp contains the highest amount of iodine than any other food on this planet. One serving of kelp contains around 2000 micrograms of iodine.

Baked Potato

Baked potatoes are another great source of iodine. A medium sized baked potato provides 60 micrograms of iodine, helping you meet 40% of the daily recommended value. Besides, the baked potato is also rich in fiber, vitamins, minerals and potassium.

Dried Seaweed

Dried seaweed is the best source of iodine. A quarter serving of dried seaweed provides a whopping 4500 micrograms of iodine. This is more than 3000% of the daily value of iodine. Make sure you consume seaweed in small portions to gain all the benefits.

Codfish

Fish extract iodine from the seawater. Cod is a delicious, moist and a low-calorie fish that comes packed with several essential nutrients like omega 3 fatty acids, protein, folate, vitamin D, E and potassium. A three-ounce serving of cod provides 99 micrograms of iodine, amounting to 99% of the daily value.

Shrimp

As mentioned earlier, seafoods are great sources of iodine and shrimp is no exception. A three-ounce serving of shrimp provides 35 micrograms of iodine, around a quarter of the recommended daily value. Besides, regular consumption of shrimp can also raise your protein, calcium and other essential mineral levels in the body.

Himalaya Crystal Sea Salt

Himalaya sea salt, also known as gray salt, is an excellent alternative to table salt. A half gram of Himalaya salt provides an incredible 250 micrograms of iodine, over 150% of the daily value of iodine. So, consume this salt in moderation.

Turkey Breast

Three ounces of turkey breast can provide 34 micrograms of iodine, around 23% of the daily value of this essential mineral. Turkey is also a good source of B complex vitamins, potassium and phosphorus, which are essential to a healthy body. Lean turkey is low in calories too, with three ounces containing just 70 calories.

Dried Prunes

Consuming five dried prunes a day can provide you with fiber, boron, vitamins, mineral and 13 micrograms of iodine. Dried prunes are a calorie dense food, and hence should be consumed in moderation.

Navy Beans

Beans are one of the most versatile foods that you can include in your diet. A half-cup serving of navy beans can provide you with protein, potassium, copper, folate, calcium and iodine. You also get around 32 micrograms of iodine with every half cup serving of navy beans.

Tuna Fish

Tuna contains high levels of iodine. Three ounces of tuna provide 17 micrograms of iodine, i.e. 11% of your daily iodine value. It also provides the body with vitamin D, iron, protein and minerals.

Boiled Eggs

A boiled egg can help you meet 12 micrograms of iodine, around 9% of the daily value. It also supplies the body with vitamin A, E, antioxidants, calcium, protein and zinc.
Enjoy a boiled egg with cottage cheese and slice it to pair with a leafy green and vegetable salad.

Yogurt

Yogurt is one of the healthiest foods to include in your daily diet. It is also an excellent option for increasing the iodine levels in your body. A cup of yogurt provides 154 micrograms of iodine and 154 calories. So, enjoy a yogurt smoothie for breakfast or combine it with berries for a light evening snack.

Bananas

Banana is an excellent energy boosting fruit. It contains a high potassium content that energizes you in a jiffy. However, not many are aware of the iodine content in bananas. A medium sized banana provides 3 micrograms of iodine, amounting to 2% of the daily value.

Strawberries

Strawberries are a nutrient dense fruit that provides the body with a plethora of essential vitamins and minerals. This delicious fruit is a surprising source of iodine as well. A cup serving of iodine contains 13 micrograms of iodine, around 10% of what an average person needs in a day.

Lobster

A 100-gram serving of lobster provides 100 micrograms of this essential mineral, around 67% of the daily value. Moreover, lobsters are quite low in fat content, making them a perfect choice for health-conscious people. Lower cholesterol levels in lobsters help to maintain the triglyceride levels, thereby keeping the heart healthy. Lobsters are also rich in omega 3 fatty acids.

Cranberries

This bright colored fruit provides a plethora of health benefits. It contains high concentrations of vitamin C, K, B, antioxidants and fiber. This fruit is an amazing source of iodine as well. Four ounces of cranberries provide 400 micrograms of iodine, equaling to 267% of the daily value. Cranberry is also renowned for its positive effects on urinary tract infection. The fruit is low in calories as well.

Green Beans
A half-cup serving of green beans can help you meet 2% of the daily value of iodine. Green beans are a great source of folate, vitamin B, C, protein and potassium as well. It provides nearly 40% of the daily value of folate and 53% of the daily value of fiber, which protects the colon and flushes the amount of toxins from it.

Pineapple
Pineapple is also a good source of iodine. It contains a range of vitamins, minerals and bromelain, an anti-inflammatory enzyme used for the treatment of autoimmune disorder. Pineapple also acts as an anticoagulant, lowering the blood pressure.

Rhubarb
Rhubarb has been used since the 3rd century BC for its medicinal properties. It is one of the best sources of iodine. In addition, it also provides calcium, manganese, copper, iron, phosphorus, and zinc. Its roots contain anthraquinone, a stimulant laxative used for relieving constipation.

Watercress
Watercress is one of the best sources of iodine for the vegans. In fact, its high iodine content gives it a nutritional breakaway value from other cruciferous vegetables. Cruciferous vegetables are also known for their anti-cancer effects. The anti-cancer benefits of watercress arise from the high levels of antioxidants present in it. Watercress also provides a wide range of vitamins and other nutrients. You can use this versatile vegetable in green salad, pasta or soups for a subtle peppery flavor.

Thyroid disease runs in my family and it has taken me a very long time to find the right doctor to work with. I highly suggest getting off synthetic thyroid pills and try Armour or Nature Thyoid are a few medications I take.

The most common thyroid problem women face is hypothyroidism, the thyroid does not make enough thyroid hormone. Without this hormone, your metabolism slows, and you may gain weight easily, feel sluggish, no energy, very emotional, and bouts of depression. I believe we are misdiagnosed and not enough research is spent on female issues, just saying.

Your periods may become irregular, dry skin and nails can also be an issue. About 10% of women have an underactive thyroid. This can be due from high iodine in the diet increases risks and/or smoking.

Your body needs iodine but cannot make it on its own. It's up to the foods we eat to provide our bodies with this necessary element. The thyroid requires iodine to synthesize hormones, and when the body does not have enough, it can lead to many serious health issues including enlarged thyroid, infertility, autoimmune disease, and increased risk of thyroid cancer.

Why is iodine deficiency a concern?
Iodine deficiency is a huge problem in some countries, especially for pregnant and breastfeeding women. Iodine is needed to make thyroid hormone, which is needed for brain development, iodine deficiency can cause brain damage in unborn babies.

When the thyroid gets inflamed, it can leak out hormone, so you become a little hyperthyroid when the gland overproduces thyroid hormone. When you run out of thyroid hormone, you may become hypothyroid until your gland heals.

Symptoms can be very subtle. Some women lose weight; others feel anxious. You might blame these things on being a new mom. But if the diagnosis is missed, it's not usually critical. If it's mild, you just watch it. The whole thing resolves within several months in most women.

If it's severe, you may need treatment for the symptoms. In most women, the hyperthyroid and hypothyroid phases last several weeks.

The Endocrine Society recommends testing if a woman has symptoms of hypothyroidism or if she has anti-thyroid antibodies, a family history of autoimmune disease or other risk factors for hypothyroidism.

How do you know if you have hypothyroidism? It's tricky, because many of the symptoms are vague and can be easily blamed on lifestyle. Fatigue, for instance, may be the result of being busy, not just an underactive thyroid. Weight gain may come from eating too much or not getting enough exercise.

You need to get a TSH test – a blood test that measures the amount of thyroid-stimulating hormone in your blood. If your thyroid isn't making enough thyroid hormone, your pituitary will make more TSH, which tells the thyroid to make more of its hormone.

How is hypothyroidism treated? You take a synthetic version of thyroid hormone in a pill to replace what your body isn't making.

Can your thyroid go in the other direction, becoming too active? Hyperthyroidism is much less common than hypothyroidism, affecting just 1% of the U.S. population. It's also more complex and difficult to diagnose and treat.

In hyperthyroidism, the thyroid is making too much thyroid hormone, which can cause shakiness, heart palpitations, insomnia and weight loss.

How do you treat hyperthyroidism?

It can be treated with anti-thyroid medications, radioactive iodine or surgery to remove the thyroid. I have done all three and it was finally removed. I had both…

Whatever you do, if you have hyper-thyroid, make sure you have an experienced doctor taking care of your needs.

You should be aware of what the front of your neck feels like. If you feel any new lumps, which could be thyroid nodules, tell your doctor. Most thyroid nodules aren't cancerous, but they still need to be checked out. They also don't always cause symptoms. Many people really have no idea they have one until a doctor feels it or it gets picked up on imaging.

So, when you have a check-up, should you ask for a TSH test? If you have symptoms of hyperthyroidism or hypothyroidism, you should have TSH, T3, T4 tested.

However, experts disagree about routine testing in people

without symptoms. It is your health and you must be honest with your doctor to share exactly how you are feeling.

My biofeedback system is very accurate when it scans your hormones. I am not a doctor, but I have the tools to educate and train you to get the proper testing so you can seek medical attention.

I highly recommend reading my Doctor's book, Dr. Hilda Maldonado, M.D. Dr. Hilda too had thyroid issues that were undiagnosed and she found her answers. Now she assists her patients daily. You can find the book below on Amazon.

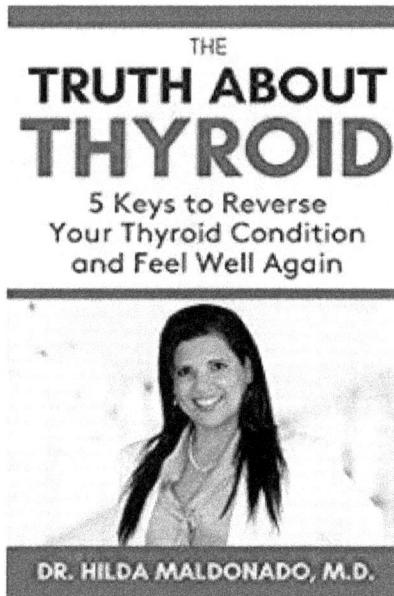

THE

TRUTH ABOUT
THYROID
5 Keys to Reverse
Your Thyroid Condition
and Feel Well Again

DR. HILDA MALDONADO, M.D.

10 OILS

I am fascinated by Essential Oils but a beginner. I have tried most brands but my personal brand is Ameo Oils. I did some research and found this article so I could share the history of Essential Oils with you.

History of Essential Oils Around the World
ARTICLE BY LEAH MORGAN, CLINICAL AROMATHERAPIST

Essential oils, or aromatic oils as they were once called, have been used by many cultures around the world for centuries. Their uses varied between cultures from religious purposes to healing the sick. It is difficult to pinpoint exactly when essential oils gained notoriety as effective healing agents, but eventually the knowledge of essential oils spread around the globe.

The earliest evidence of human knowledge of the healing properties of plants was found in Lascaux, located in the Dordogne region in France. There, cave paintings suggest the use of medicinal plants in everyday life that have been carbon dated as far back as 18,000 B.C.E.

Egypt
Evidence and recorded history have both shown that the Egyptians used aromatic oils as early as 4500 B.C.E. They became renowned for their knowledge of cosmetology, ointments and aromatic oils. The most famous of their

herbal preparations "Kyphi" was a mixture of 16 ingredients that could be used as incense, perfume or medicine.

They used balsams, perfumed oils, scented barks, resins, spices and aromatic vinegars in everyday life. Oils and pastes from plants were transformed into pills, powders, suppositories, medicinal cakes and ointments.

Ashes and smoke from aniseed, cedar, onion, garlic, grapes and watermelon among others were also used. At the height of Egypt's power, priests were the only authorities allowed to use aromatic oils, as they were regarded as necessary to be at one with the gods.

Specific fragrances were dedicated to each deity and their statues were anointed with these oils by their followers. Pharaohs had their own special blends for meditation, love, war and so on.

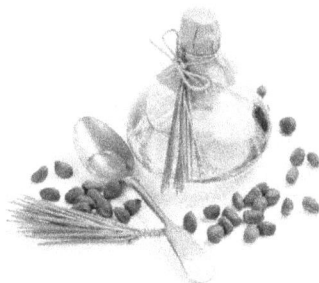

Aromatic gums such as cedar and myrrh were used in the embalming process and traces of these have been found on mummies today. Despite the importance of aromatic oils in Egyptian society, they never distilled their own and in fact imported oils of cypress and cedar.

China

The use of aromatic oils was first recorded in China between 2697-2597 B.C.E during the reign of Huang Ti, the legendary Yellow Emperor. His famous book "The Yellow Emperor's Book of Internal Medicine" contains uses for several aromatics and is still considered a useful classic by practitioners of eastern medicine today.

India

Traditional Indian medicine called "Ayur Veda" has a 3000-year history of incorporating essential oils into their healing potions. Vedic literature lists over 700 substances including cinnamon, ginger, myrrh and sandalwood as effective for healing.

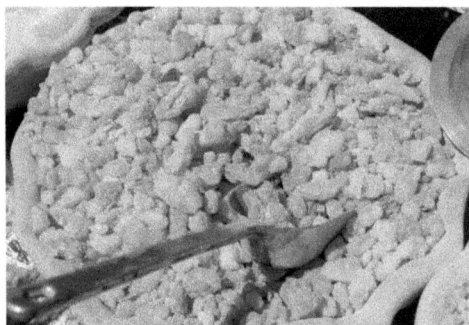

During the outbreak of the Bubonic Plague, Ayurveda was used successfully in replacing ineffective antibiotics. The purpose of aromatic plants and oils were not only for medicinal purposes, but were believed to be a Godly part of nature and played an integral role to the spiritual and philosophical outlook in Ayurvedic medicine.

Greece

Between 400-500 B.C.E. the Greeks recorded knowledge of essential oils adopted from the Egyptians. Ointment of Myrrh was carried by soldiers into battle to counter infections.

The Greek physician Hypocrites (460-377 B.C.E.), known to us as the "Father of Medicine" documented the effects of some 300 plants including thyme, saffron, marjoram, cumin and peppermint.

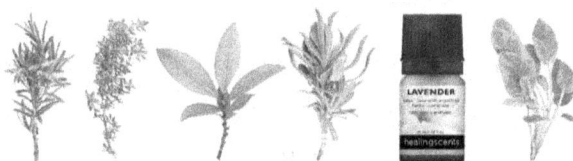

Hypocrites' extensive knowledge of plants and their essences was Ayurvedic in origin and was gained in part through the Greek soldiers' encounters with Ayurvedic medicine on the Indian sub-continent during their travels with Alexander the Great. They found Ayurveda to be harmonious with their own medicinal practices and evidence of the mingling of these two traditions can still be found in use by remote tribes today.

Hypocrites wrote "a perfumed bath and a scented massage daily is the way to good health." The literature left by him and his students contains the most important principle in modern medicine; "Above all the purpose of a doctor is to awaken the natural healing energies within the body". Hypocrites' wisdom influences modern medicine to this day in the form of the "Hippocratic Oath" taken by all doctors.

Galen was another Greek whose reportedly vast knowledge of plants and their medicines had a remarkable impact on how we classify information today. He began as a surgeon at a school for gladiators and it was said that no gladiator died of his wounds during Galen's term as physician. His reputation became known and he was promoted to personal physician to the Roman Emperor, Marcus Aurelius. He wrote a great deal on the theory of plant medicine and divided plants into various medicinal categories that are still known as "Galenic" today.

Rome
The Romans were known for lavishly applying perfumed oil to their bodies, bedding and clothes. It was also customary for the Romans to use oils in massage and baths. Roman physicians brought books written by Galen and Hypocrites with them as they fled during the fall of the Roman Empire; these texts were later translated into Persian, Arabic and other languages.

Persia
Ali-Ibn Sana (commonly known as Avicenna the Arab) lived from 980 -1037 A.D. He was a child prodigy and became a well-educated physician by the age of 12. Ali-Ibn wrote books on the properties of 800 plants and their effects on the human body. He is also credited for being the first person to discover and record the method of distilling essential oils. His methods are still in use.

Europe
During the Crusades, the Knights and their armies were responsible for passing on knowledge of herbal medicines that they learned in the Middle East, throughout Western

Europe. The knights acquired knowledge of distillation and carried perfumes with them.

Frankincense and pine were burned in the streets to ward off "evil spirits" during the Bubonic Plague of the 14th Century. It was noted that less people died of the plague in the areas where this was done.

In 1653 Nicholas Culpeper wrote his" The Complete Herbal" which still stands as a valuable reference. His book describes many conditions and their remedies that are still appropriate today.

French Chemist René-Maurice Gattefossé coined the term "Aromatherapy" while investigating the antiseptic properties of essential oils. Gattefosse's book "Aromatherapy" was published in 1928 in which he details cases of essential oils and their healing capabilities. The book was influential in medical practices in France.

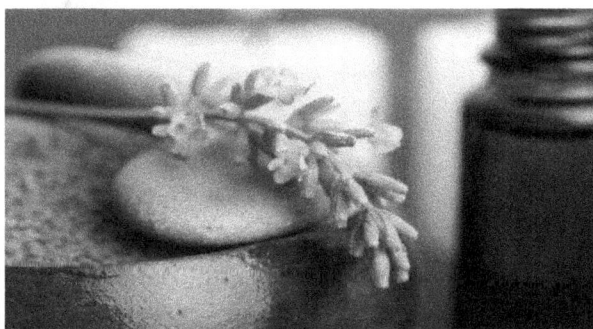

Gattefossé discovered the incredible healing properties of Lavender accidentally when a small explosion occurred in his laboratory. One of Gattefossé's hands was badly burned. He quickly immersed it in the nearest tray of liquid. The liquid was essential oil of lavender and to his astonishment

Gattefossé observed that his hand healed with no infection or scarring.

Gattefossé and a colleague conducted further research on the healing properties of lavender and introduced it to many of the hospitals in France. During the outbreak of Spanish influenza there were no reported deaths of hospital personnel, which was credited to the use of lavender.

*****

This History of Essential Oils article was shared from the internet and for educational purposes. I have been using oils personally for 5 years. I diffuse them in the house, clean my floors and house with them, make my own tinctures to carry, and believe in them 100%.

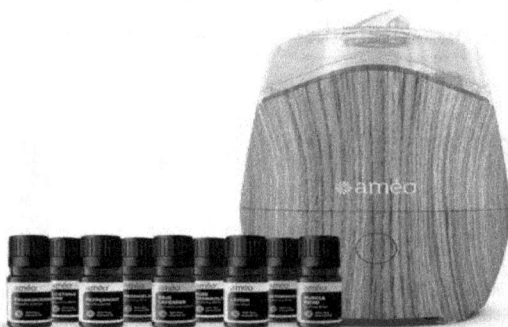

I have used many oils from Young Living, Doterra, and NOW. However, hooked on Ameo Oils due to their proprietary blends and therapeutic grade created by
Dr. Joshua Plant who sits on the Natural Institute of Health Board (NIH).

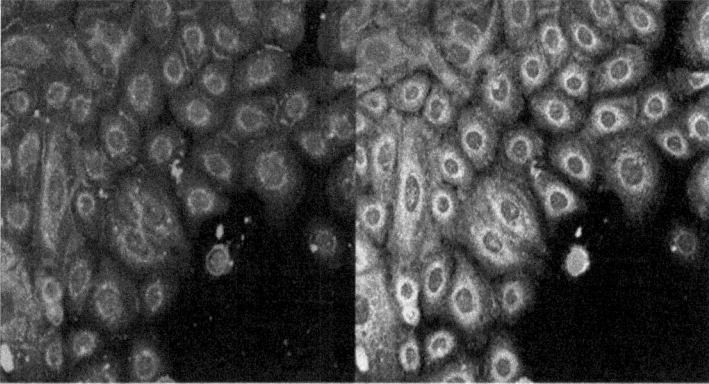

Using confocal fluorescence microscopy, we visualize living human cells and subcellular organelles both before and after exposure to Améo Essential Oils.

I recommend that my Clients test drive a few oils that they would benefit from. I believe every home should have an essential oil arsenal. They travel well, diffuse in car, diffuse in home, great to eliminate cooking odors, disinfect and clean floors and counter tops, carry in purse, and men can carry in pockets.

When I feel allergens or not my best I will put a few drops in my mouth or my water glass and presto whatever it was disappears in hours. No wonder why Frankincense and Myrrh are in the bible! They are truly my MIRACLE OILS!

A few photos below when travelling in Venice, Italy I gave a few of my first edition of my book away and they were kind enough to let me take their pictures.

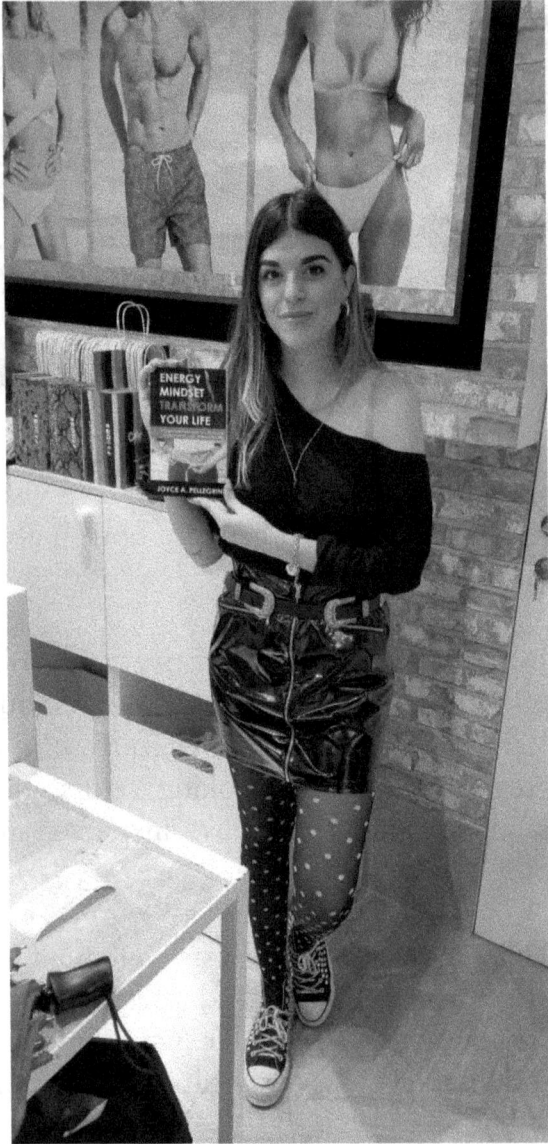

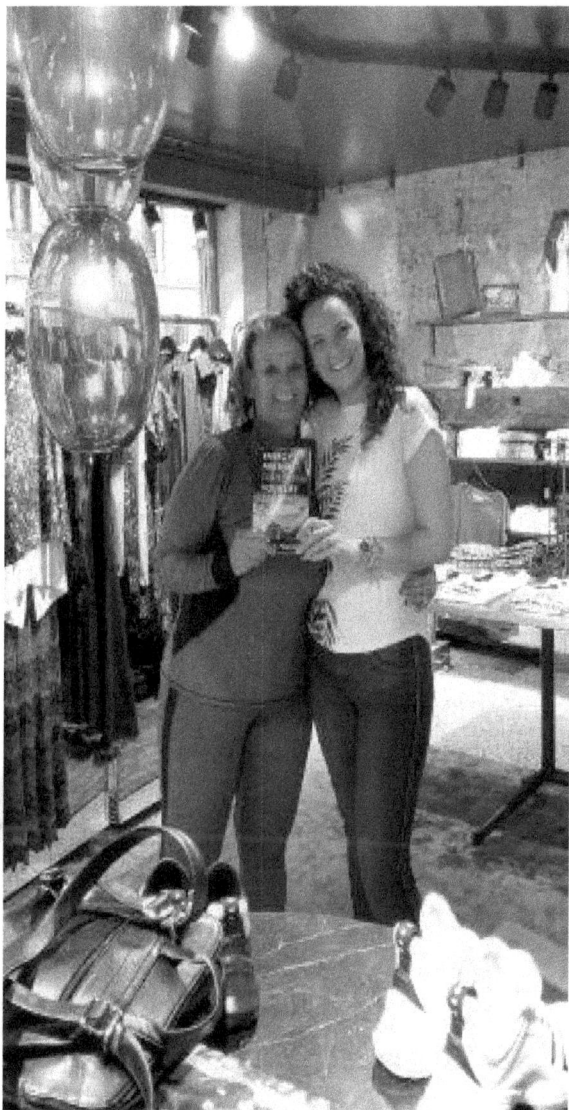

ABOUT THE AUTHOR

Joyce Pellegrini has been passionate about health and wellness since she left corporate America in 2001. Through her journey to destress her life, mind, body, and spirit using a holistic approach to health. She only shares what she has tried which has worked for her.

From feeling dead inside, suicidal, depressed, and totally alone to being at the top of her game. Her mission in life is to motivate others to take control of their stress filled life and take their personal power back! The goal is to inspire you to act now before it is too late. Don't let the EMT's take you away before your time.

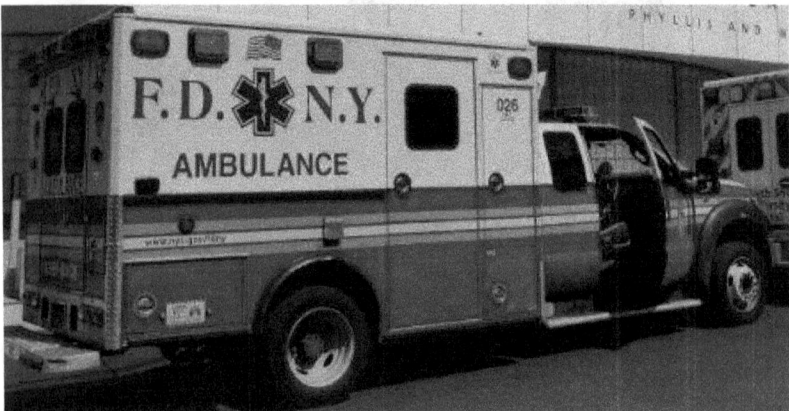

This life is not a dress rehearsal. No one will ever make you healthy or happy. It is up to you with families like yours to lead the natural health revolution.

Isn't it time to live life by design and not by default?

LET'S DO THIS!

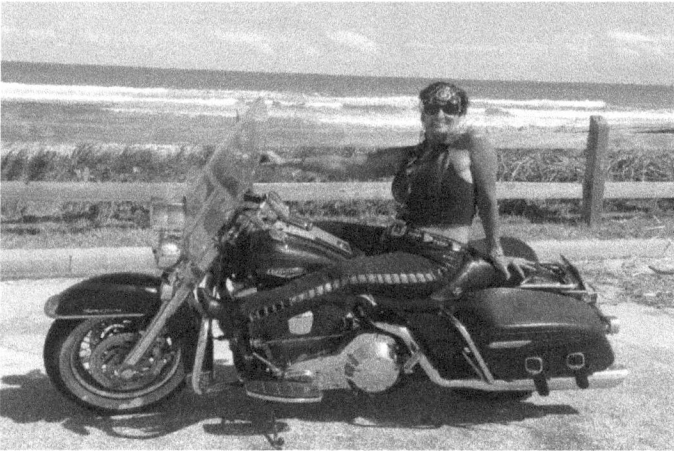

Joyce Pellegrini
LIVE YOUR LIFE FULL THROTTLE!

For More Info
www.EMTYourLife.com

www.ingramcontent.com/pod-product-compliance
Lightning Source LLC
Chambersburg PA
CBHW072206270326
41930CB00011B/2556